OPCS Surveys of Psychiatric
Morbidity in Great Britain

Report 5

Physical complaints, service use and treatment of residents with psychiatric disorders

Howard Meltzer

Baljit Gill

Mark Petticrew

Kerstin Hinds

London: HMSO

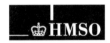

Published by HMSO and available from:

HMSO Publications Centre
(Mail, fax and telephone orders only)
PO Box 276, London SW8 5DT
Telephone orders 0171 873 9090
General enquiries 0171 873 0011
(queuing system in operation for both numbers)
Fax orders 0171 873 8200

HMSO Bookshops
49 High Holborn, London WC1V 6HB
(counter service only)
0171 873 0011 Fax 0171 831 1326
68–69 Bull Street, Birmingham B4 6AD
0121 236 9696   Fax 0121 236 9699
33 Wine Street, Bristol BS1 2BQ
0117 9264306 Fax 0117 9294515
9–21 Princess Street, Manchester M60 8AS
0161 834 7201 Fax 0161 833 0634
16 Arthur Street, Belfast BT1 4GD
01232 238451 Fax 01232 235401
71 Lothian Road, Edinburgh EH3 9AZ
0131 228 4181 Fax 0131 229 2734
The HMSO Oriel Bookshop
The Friary, Cardiff CF1 4AA
01222 395548 Fax 01222 384347

HMSO's Accredited Agents
(see Yellow Pages)

and through good booksellers

Authors' acknowledgements

We would like to thank everybody who contributed to the survey and the production of this report. Administrators, medical, nursing and support staff in the establishments we visited were of great assistance to the OPCS interviewers not only in organising contact with respondents but helping as proxy informants when subjects could not manage an interview.

We were supported by our specialist colleagues in OPCS who carried out the sampling, fieldwork, coding and editing stages.

The project was steered by a group comprising the following, to whom thanks are due for assistance and specialist advice at various stages of the survey:

Department of Health:
Dr Rachel Jenkins (chair)
Dr Elaine Gadd
Ms Val Roberts
Ms Antonia Roberts

Psychiatric epidemiologists:
Professor Paul Bebbington
Dr Terry Brugha
Professor Glyn Lewis
Dr Mike Farrell
Dr Jacquie de Alarcon

Office of Population Censuses and Surveys:
Ms Jil Matheson
Dr Howard Meltzer
Ms Baljit Gill
Dr Mark Petticrew
Ms Kerstin Hinds

Most importantly, we would like to thank all the participants in the survey for their cooperation.

Contents

List of tables

Notes

1 Tables showing percentages
The row or column percentages may add to 99% or 101% because of rounding.

The varying positions of the percentage signs and bases in the tables denote the presentation of different types of information. Where there is a percentage sign at the head of a column and the base at the foot, the whole distribution is presented and the individual percentages add to between 99% and 101%. Where there is no percentage sign in the table and a note above the figures, the figures refer to the proportion of people who had the attribute being discussed, and the complementary proportion, to add to 100%, is not shown in the table.

Standard errors are shown in brackets beside percentages in the tables.

The following conventions have been used within tables showing percentages:
-       no cases
0   values less than 0.5%

2 Small bases
Very small bases have been avoided wherever possible because of the relatively high sampling errors that attach to small numbers. Often where the numbers are not large enough to justify the use of all categories, classifications have been condensed. However, an item within a classification is occasionally shown separately, even though the base is small, because to combine it with another large category would detract from the value of the larger category. In general, percentage distributions are shown if the base is 30 or more. Where the base is slightly lower, actual numbers are shown in square brackets

3 Significant differences
The bases for some sub-groups presented in the tables were small such that the standard errors around estimates for these groups are biased. Confidence intervals which take account of these biased standard errors were calculated and, although they are not presented in the tables, they were used in testing for statistically significant differences. Statistical significance is explained in Appendix B to this Report.

Focus of the report and survey definitions

Focus of the report

This report is the second of three to look at data from the OPCS survey of psychiatric morbidity among residents of institutions.[1] It presents results about adults living in hospitals, residential care homes and other types of residential accommodation; institutions whose primary purpose is the long term care of people with mental health disorders. People with mental disorders who were temporary residents of institutions, such as those in acute, short-stay NHS hospital facilities were excluded from the survey.

Coverage of institutions

Although a fairly detailed classification of types of institutions was made during data collection, five main types of institution have been used for analysis.

Because there are often different definitions of the degree of supervision in residential accommodation, descriptions of what constituted non-supervised, supervised and highly supervised accommodation were included in the questionnaires with the aim of obtaining a consistent assessment among interviewers.

Ordinary housing or recognised lodging

Unsupervised in ordinary housing with a degree of protection, eg from eviction if in rent arrears.

Supervised in ordinary housing with regular domiciliary supervision of personal care, household maintenance, hygiene safety and rent payments.

Recognised lodging where the landlady has been selected for qualities of kindness and standard of care. Supervises personal care, hygiene, and rent payments.

Group homes

Unsupervised group home where a group of people live together in an ordinary house, with protected rent and occasional visits.

Supervised group home where a group of people live together in an ordinary house but have regular (up to daily) visits by housekeeper for household maintenance. No care staff live in.

Clustered group homes where a warden lives nearby and makes regular domiciliary checks. Some are built around a quadrangle with the entrance by the warden's flat.

Hostels

Supervised hostel where care staff live in and are on call at night. Provide regular domiciliary supervision.

Higher supervision hostel where care staff are in attendance all night.

Intensive supervision hostel with higher staff levels than above. For people with severe behaviour disturbance or disability.

Coverage of residents

Only **permanent residents** aged 16-64 were covered in the survey. A permanent resident was defined as:

- living in the sampled institution for the past six months;

- living in the sampled institution for less than 6 months but:

  - had been living in residential

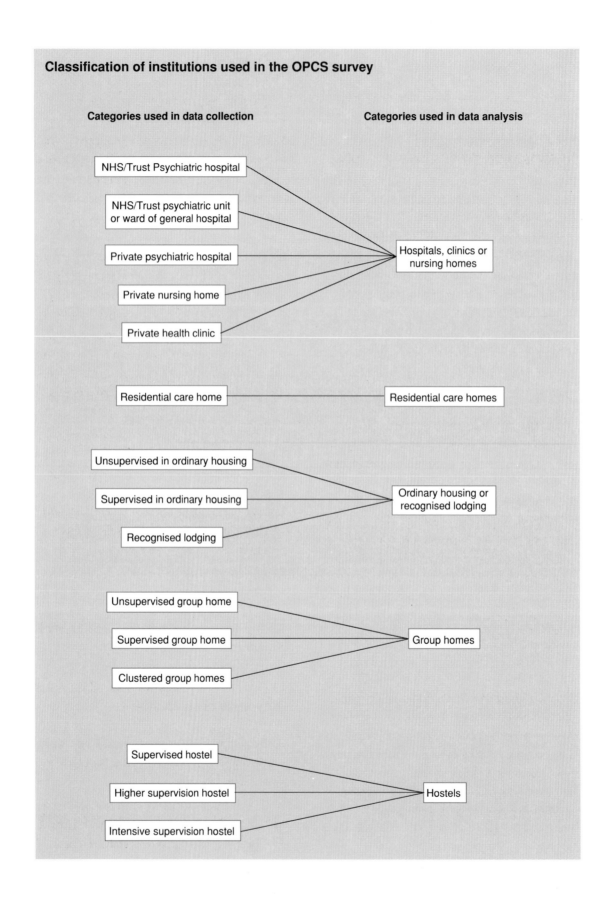

Classification of institutions used in the OPCS survey

Categories used in data collection

Categories used in data analysis

NHS/Trust Psychiatric hospital

NHS/Trust psychiatric unit or ward of general hospital

Private psychiatric hospital

Private nursing home

Private health clinic

Hospitals, clinics or nursing homes

Residential care home

Residential care homes

Unsupervised in ordinary housing

Supervised in ordinary housing

Recognised lodging

Ordinary housing or recognised lodging

Unsupervised group home

Supervised group home

Clustered group homes

Group homes

Supervised hostel

Higher supervision hostel

Intensive supervision hostel

Hostels

accommodation for the past six months, or

- had no other permanent address, or
- was likely to stay in the institution for the foreseeable future.

Coverage and classification of mental disorders

In this report, we only consider residents who had one of the following three general categories of mental disorder:

- Schizophrenia, delusional or schizo affective disorders

- Affective psychoses (mania and bipolar affective disorder)

- Neurotic disorders (Generalised Anxiety Disorder, depressive episode, mixed anxiety and depressive disorder, phobia, Obsessive-Compulsive Disorder, panic)

The approach used to assess psychotic psychopathology was to ask OPCS interviewers to find out from residents or staff information about clinical assessment and treatments by:

- asking residents directly what was the matter with them;

- asking staff, what was the matter with the subject, (if the subject could not answer but gave informed consent for another person to do so);

- asking residents or carers whether subjects were taking anti-psychotic drugs or having anti-psychotic injections;

- establishing whether residents had contact with any health care professional for a mental, nervous or emotional problem labelled as a psychotic illness.

The Clinical Interview Schedule (CIS-R) was used to identify neurotic disorders.[2] It establishes the existence of a particular neurotic symptom in the past month and leads the interviewer on to further enquiry giving a more detailed assessment of the symptom **in the past week**: frequency, duration, severity and time since onset. Algorithms are applied to the data to arrive at a classification of six types of neurotic disorder.

The few residents identified (by self-report or staff-report) as having an organic mental disorder (2%), mental and behavioural disorders due to psychoactive substance abuse (1%), behavioural syndromes associated with psychological disturbances and physical factors (1%) or disorders of psychological development (1%) are excluded from consideration in this report.

Because of the absence of clinical research assessments for diagnostic classification, eg SCAN, care has to be taken in making comparisons of results presented in this report with those from the private household survey and other surveys among residents of institutions.

Coverage of the report

In this report we investigate:

- the relationship between the physical and mental health of residents

- medication and other forms of treatment received by residents at their own and other establishments

- the use of services received by residents at their own and other establishments

All three factors are considered for each of the three main categories of disorder and where appropriate by type of institution.

Other reports on the institution survey

Report 4

Report 4 presents the prevalence of mental disorders in the institutional population. It shows that prevalence of disorders (based on ICD-10 chapters) varies according to type of institution. Two tables from this report showing the proportions of residents with each type of disorder by type of institution are shown below.

Report 4 also includes information on the survey methodology: the sample design, response, and the method used to weight the data. The questionnaires used in the survey are printed as an Appendix to Report 4.

Report 6

Report 6 looks at the same three groups of residents as this report but focuses on their economic activity and social functioning. This includes difficulties associated with mental disorders in respect of activities of daily living, employment, perceived social support and finances. Information is also presented on and the use of tobacco, alcohol and drugs.

Proportions of residents with each type of disorder by type of hospital setting

		NHS psychiatric hospital	NHS unit/ward of general hospital	Private hospital, clinic or nursing home	All hospitals, clinics, or nursing homes
Primary diagnosis (based on ICD-10)		%	%	%	%
F00-F09	Organic mental disorders	4	1	1	2
F10-F19	Mental and behavioural disorders due to psychoactive substance use	0	0	0	0
F20-F29	Schizophrenia, delusional and schizoaffective disorders	75	81	61	72
F30-F39	Mood disorders excluding depressive episode: affective psychoses	7	10	24	14
F40-F48	Neurotic, stress-related and somatoform disorders including depressive episode	4	3	4	4
F50-F59	Behavioural syndromes associated with psychological disturbances and physical factors	0	2	5	2
F60-F69	Disorders of adult personality and behaviour	1	0	0	0
F70-F79	Mental retardation	0	0	0	0
F80-F89	Disorders of psychological development	0	0	3	1
F90-F98	Behavioural and emotional disorders with onset usually occurring in childhood and adolescence	0	0	0	0
	Insufficient information	6	3	0	3
	No answer / refusal	1	0	1	0
Base (all residents)		*341*	*66*	*80*	*487*

Proportions of residents with each type of disorder by type of residential accommodation

		Residential care home	Group home	Hostels	Ordinary/ recognised housing	All residential accommodation
Primary diagnosis (based on ICD-10)		%	%	%	%	%
F00-F09	Organic mental disorders	1	0	0	0	0
F10-F19	Mental and behavioural disorders due to psychoactive substance use	1	1	0	2	1
F20-F29	Schizophrenia, delusional and schizoaffective disorders	65	68	58	76	67
F30-F39	Mood disorders excluding depressive episode: affective psychoses	7	9	3	6	6
F40-F48	Neurotic, stress-related and somatoform disorders including depressive episode	11	11	19	7	12
F50-F59	Behavioural syndromes associated with psychological disturbances and physical factors	1	0	0	0	0
F60-F69	Disorders of adult personality and behaviour	1	1	0	0	0
F70-F79	Mental retardation	0	0	0	0	0
F80-F89	Disorders of psychological development	2	0	2	2	2
F90-F98	Behavioural and emotional disorders with onset usually occurring in childhood and adolescence	0	0	0	0	0
	Insufficient information	10	8	16	6	10
	No answer / refusal	1	3	2	1	2
Base (all residents)		*297*	*166*	*125*	*94*	*705*

Notes and references

1 The institutional survey involved interviews with about 1200 randomly sampled residents in Great Britain. In addition to this survey, interviews were also conducted in private households and accommodation specifically catering for homeless people.

2 Lewis, G., Pelosi, A.J. and Dunn, G., (1992) Measuring psychiatric disorder in the community: a standardized assessment for use by lay interviewers, *Psychological Medicine*, **22**, 465-486

Summary of main findings

In 1994, 70% of adults aged 16-64 permanently resident in institutions in Great Britain that cater for people with mental health problems suffered from schizophrenia, delusional and schizoaffective disorders. About 8% suffered from affective psychosis (mainly bipolar affective disorder), 8% had neurotic disorders, and 5% had other mental disorders. For the remaining 9% there was insufficient information to categorise residents.

Each of the three chapters in this Report is devoted to a particular group of residents: those with schizophrenia, delusional or schizoaffective disorders (Chapter 1); residents who have affective psychosis (Chapter 2), and those classified as having a neurotic disorder (Chapter 3). In this Summary, the first three sections show, for each group, the main differences in the personal characteristics of residents, the treatment they received and their use of services by type of institution. In the final part of this Summary, data from all three chapters are brought together to compare the characteristics of residents by type of disorder.

Residents with schizophrenia

- Just under three quarters of all residents who had schizophrenia were men.

- The mean length of present stay in hospital was twice that in residential care homes (7.2 years compared with 3.6 years).

- Fatigue was the most prevalent neurotic symptom affecting 43% of residents with schizophrenia who were CIS-R respondents.

- Among 55-64 year olds with schizophrenia, 18% of hospital patients reported a long standing physical complaint compared with 36% of those living in any type of residential accommodation.

- The proportions of residents given antipsychotic medication ranged from 98% among hospital residents to 90% of occupants of residential care homes.

- Three factors at least doubled the odds of residents' non-compliance with taking antipsychotic medication: being aged 16-34 (cf 55-64), having A-level or higher qualifications (cf no qualifications) and living in unsupervised rather than supervised accommodation.

- Those living in ordinary housing or recognised lodgings were most likely to consult their GP for a physical complaint, 17%, and least likely to see their GP for a mental health problem, 9%.

- Overall, 8 in 10 residents with schizophrenia living in residential accommodation had at least one domiciliary visit in the past 12 months.

Residents with affective psychoses

- A quarter of all residents were divorced.

- 20% of hospital residents had been in hospital for at least ten years.

- A quarter of male residents with affective psychosis said they had epilepsy.

- About 8 in 10 were reported to be on drugs used in treating psychosis and related conditions with about half this group taking antimanic drugs. About 3 in 10 were taking antidepressants.

- Out-patient visits, made by 6 in 10 of those living in residential accommodation, were largely for treatment or check-ups relating to their mental disorder.

Residents with neurotic disorders

- The mean length of stay of the neurotic group was 2.2 years compared with 5.3 years for those with schizophrenia.

- Half the sample had Generalised Anxiety Disorder, just over a quarter had phobia or mixed anxiety and depressive disorder.

- Musculo-skeletal problems, affecting 1 in 5 of residents, were most commonly reported, predominantly arthritis and rheumatism among women and those aged 40 or over.

- Antidepressants rather than antipsychotic drugs were the most commonly reported drugs taken by those who had a neurotic disorder.

- Forty five percent of the neurotic group sometimes did not take their drugs, and twenty one percent sometimes took more than the stated dose.

- 84% of those living in residential accommodation had consulted their GP in the past 12 months.

Personal characteristics by type of disorder

The biographical profile of residents with schizophrenia, was significantly different to that of those who had an affective disorder or a neurotic disorder. Residents suffering from schizophrenia had the largest proportion of young, single men with no educational qualifications. Nevertheless, 1 in 6 schizophrenic residents had spent more than 10 years in their present institutions which were more likely to be hospitals than

Summary Table 1 Summary of personal characteristics by type of disorder

	Schizophrenia, delusional or schizoaffective disorders	Affective psychoses	Neurotic disorders
	Proportion of residents who were...		
Men	71%	58%	61%
Aged 16-24	6%	12%	21%
Single	80%	65%	65%
Divorced	13%	24%	19%
No qualifications	72%	58%	51%
In accommodation for 10 years or more	16%	9%	1%
Had a long standing physical illness	23%	42%	50%
Base	*828*	*96*	*101*

residential accommodation. Hardly any resident with a neurotic disorder had spent more than ten years in their present accommodation, which for 80% of them, was some sort of residential facility.

Half the residents with a neurotic disorder reported having a longstanding physical complaint, twice the proportion identified among those with schizophrenia.

Treatment by type of disorder

Not surprisingly the use of specific categories of drugs was associated with particular types of disorder. Nearly all residents with schizophrenia were on antipsychotic drugs, or depot injections or antimanic drugs, and about 6 in 10 were also taking anticholinergic drugs. About four-fifths of residents with affective psychosis were on drugs used in psychosis and related conditions and just over a quarter took antidepressants.

The group of residents with neurotic disorders had the largest proportion of antidepressants takers, 44%, approximately one and a half times the proportion among those with affective psychosis and nearly three times the level among the schizophrenic sample. Residents with neurotic disorders were the least compliant with their medicinal regimes; just less than half sometimes did not take their drugs compared with one in six of all other residents. Similarly, 1 in 5 of the neurotic sample sometimes took more than their stated dose, compared with 1 in 20 residents with schizophrenia or affective psychosis.

Two factors which had a marked affect on compliance were the educational attainment of residents and the degree of supervision in their institutions. Residents with neurosis who had some qualifications and were living in unsupervised lodgings or group homes were less likely than other residents to adhere to their medicinal regimes.

Summary Table 2 Summary of treatment by type of disorder

	Schizophrenia, delusional or schizoaffective disorders	Affective psychoses	Neurotic disorders
Proportion of residents taking each type of drug...			
Drugs used in psychoses and related conditions	94%	79%	35%
Antidepressants	16%	28%	44%
Hypnotics and anxiolytics	17%	23%	21%
Anticholinergic drugs	59%	40%	12%
Any CNS drugs	96%	94%	68%
Therapy or counselling	23%	28%	29%
Percentage of residents who...			
Sometimes did not take their drugs	16%	17%	45%
Sometimes took more than normal dose	5%	6%	21%
Previously had a different treatment	56%	59%	63%
Refused alternative treatment	11%	13%	12%
Base	*828*	*96*	*101*

Service use by type of disorder

Among those living in residential accommodation there were no significant differences by type of disorder in the proportions who had contacted GPs, or had been an in-patient or an out-patient in the past 12 months. The factors which increased the likelihood of contact with services were being female, having a physical complaint and living in unsupervised rather than supervised accommodation.

The main difference in service use by type of disorder was that compared with the neurotic group, residents with schizophrenia were more likely to have turned down help or support in the past 12 months despite being more likely to seek help.

Summary Table 3 Summary of service use by type of disorder (among those living in residential accommodation)

	Schizophrenia, delusional or schizoaffective disorders	Affective psychoses	Neurotic disorders
Proportion of residents who...			
Consulted GP in past 2 weeks	22%	27%	34%
Consulted GP in past 12 months	76%	78%	84%
Had an in-patient stay in past 12 months	6%	14%	13%
Had an out-patient visit in past 12 months	56%	58%	59%
Had any type of domiciliary visit in past 12 months	79%	78%	62%
Turned down help or support in past 12 months	10%	13%	3%
Decided not to seek professional help when felt they need it	10%	12%	21%
Base	*470*	*45*	*81*

1   Residents with schizophrenia, delusional or schizoaffective disorders

1.1 Introduction

This chapter focuses on those residents living in institutions who had schizophrenia, delusional or schizoaffective disorders, classified by self report or by diagnoses given by staff. Because no clinical assessment was made by the interviewing team in arriving at this broad diagnostic category, residents could not be further classified as having either schizophrenia, a delusional disorder or a schizoaffective disorder.[1] Although interviewers carried out a CIS-R interview, this does not cover psychosis; SCAN interviews were not carried out in the institutions survey.

In this chapter, the term, residents with schizophrenia, is used as a shorthand description of the 828 adults classified as suffering from schizophrenia, delusional or schizoaffective disorders.

1.2 Descriptive profile of residents

Personal characteristics

Just under three quarters of all residents who had schizophrenia were men. Their average age was in the mid-forties and for the most part they were single, white men who had not obtained any educational qualifications. The profile for women was similar to men in terms of their age distribution, ethnicity and educational attainment. However, women with schizophrenia were less likely than their male counterparts to be single (66% compared with 86%) and twice as likely to be divorced (21% compared with 10%).

Schizophrenics who resided in hospitals had a slightly different socio-demographic profile than those living in residential facilities in relation to age and educational qualifications. In psychiatric wards, units or hospitals there were more residents aged 16-34 and more residents without any educational qualifications. These two factors, age and educational attainment, come up repeatedly in later sections of this chapter as being associated with variations in residents' behaviour, for example, in their compliance with medicinal regimes or use of services. (*Tables 1.1 to 1.4*)

Institutional characteristics

The mean length of time residents with schizophrenia had been living at their present establishment was 5.3 years. It should be noted that to be included in the survey, residents had to have spent the past 6 months in any type of residential accommodation. The mean length of stay in hospital was twice that in residential care homes (7.2 years compared with 3.6 years). However, the median length of stay in both types of accommodation was the same, 2.5 years. This is a reflection of the fact that 1 in 8 hospital residents with schizophrenia had been in psychiatric facilities for at least 20 years. The survey did not identify any residents in residential care homes, or in group homes or hostels, who had been there so long. The use of small residential facilities in the community to house adults with psychiatric disorders is a policy which has developed over the past two or three decades.

Adults with schizophrenia who were residents of hospitals, clinics or nursing homes came to their present accommodation mostly from their own homes (45%) or from another hospital (38%).

Similarly, many of those living in residential

accommodation also came directly from hospital: almost a half of those now living in supported accommodation (ordinary/ recognised lodging) and a third of those living in group homes or hostels. However, a sizeable proportion of residents moved between group homes, hostels and supported accommodation. For example, a quarter of adults with schizophrenia living in supported housing or recognised lodging were in a similar sort of accommodation at their previous address. One in six of those living in a residential care home had come from another residential care home. (*Table 1.5*)

Psychiatric characteristics

All residents who could manage an interview were asked the revised version of the Clinical Interview Schedule (CIS-R). This was to look at neurotic symptomatology, even for those eventually classified as having schizophrenia, delusional or schizoaffective disorders. Of the 828 residents with schizophrenia, 72% managed to answer the questions in the CIS-R. When diagnostic algorithms were applied to their responses, neurotic disorders were identified for a third of those living in supported accommodation, about a half of group home and hostel residents and a half of those living in hospitals.[2]

Fatigue was the most prevalent neurotic symptom affecting 43% of CIS-R respondents. About a third had sleep problems, worry or anxiety, and a quarter had significant symptoms of depression, depressive ideas and problems with concentration. The most prevalent neurotic disorder was General Anxiety Disorder, affecting 22% of all the schizophrenic residents who had answered the CIS-R. (*Table 1.6*)

1.3   Physical complaints

About a quarter of all residents with schizophrenia had a physical complaint. The

most frequently mentioned problems were musculo-skeletal complaints (6%) nervous system complaints (6%) and endocrine, nutritional or metabolic diseases (5%). The prevalence of physical complaints increased with age and were most commonly reported among 55-64 year old women: 18% suffered from musculo-skeletal complaints, 15% had heart and circulatory system complaints, and 10% stated they had a complaint related to the digestive system. Among all 55-64 year olds, that is, both men and women with schizophrenia, the proportion in hospital who reported a long standing physical complaint was half that of those living in any type of residential accommodation, 18% compared with 36%. (*Tables 1.7 to 1.9*)

1.4   Treatment

At least nine out of ten residents with schizophrenia were on drugs classified by the British National Formulary as "drugs used in psychosis and related conditions". This includes depot injections as well as antipsychotic and antimanic drugs. The proportions of residents given any of these drugs ranged from 98% among hospital residents to 90% of occupants of residential care homes. Because so many residents were on "drug cocktails", for example, an antipsychotic drug plus depot injections plus anticholinergic and antiepileptic drugs to relieve side effects, there may have been omissions in reporting some of the drugs used in treating psychosis.

Among residents with schizophrenia who had a CIS-R interview, 18% reported being on antidepressants and 16% on hypnotics and anxiolytics. Those identified as having a neurotic disorder were twice as likely as schizophrenic residents without a neurotic disorder to be on these drugs: 24% compared with 14% for antidepressants and 21% compared with 12% for hypnotics and anxiolytics. This may help to explain marked differences in the use of these drugs by type of institution. For instance 24% of residents of residential care homes were taking anxiolytics and hypnotics compared with 8% of residents with schizophrenia living in group homes or supported accommodation. Similarly, about 1 in 5 of those living in residential care homes, hostels, and supported accommodation were on antidepressants compared with 1 in 10 residents of hospitals and group homes. (*Tables 1.10 to 1.11*)

Residents with schizophrenia were asked whether they sometimes did not take their medication even though they knew they should. One in six answered "yes". Three factors at least doubled the odds of residents' non-compliance with taking antipsychotic medication: being aged 16-34 (cf 55-64), having A-level or higher qualifications (cf no qualifications) and living in unsupervised rather than supervised accommodation. Unsupervised accommodation refers to unstaffed group homes and unsupervised supported accommodation or recognised housing. Although residents from ethnic minorities have been regarded as less compliant, the results from this survey do not support this contention. Among those who were non-compliant with their medicinal regimes, a half said they had not taken their antipsychotic medication within the past week. When asked why they did not take their drugs, the most frequently stated reasons were dislike of taking medication (29%) or simply forgot (28%). (*Tables 1.12 to 1.14*)

Some residents, about 5%, sometimes took more than their stated dose. This behaviour was most prevalent among 35-44 year olds, those with the highest educational qualifications, residents of group homes, hostels and recognised lodging, and most noticeably among unsupervised residents, 23%. (*Tables 1.15 to 1.16*)

Just over half the residents with schizophrenia,

56%, had previously been given a different treatment from that which were getting at the moment and this proportion hardly varied by socio-demographic or institutional characteristics. The change in treatment was either a different drug or a different method of administration; going from oral medication to injections or vice versa. Practically all those who had a previous treatment, 95%, had stopped their previous treatment and started a new one on professional advice. (*Table 1.17*)

When asked about refusing other forms of treatment, 1 in 9 residents said that they had, mostly not wanting to change the drugs they were taking for another one or not wanting to change to injections from oral medication. Again, the most highly educated individuals were those most likely to refuse alternative treatment. (*Table 1.18*)

1.5 Use of services

To examine the use of services, residents with schizophrenia living in residential accommodation are separated from those living in hospitals and nursing homes as the services available at these two types of institutions vary considerably. For those living in residential accommodation five types of service contact were investigated:

- Consulted GP in past 2 weeks
- Consulted GP in past 12 months
- Had an in-patient stay in the past 12 months
- Had an out-patient visit in the past 12 months
- Had a domiciliary visit in the past 12 months

For hospital residents, the service arrangements considered were:

- Services received at own hospital
- In-patient stays at other hospitals
- Out-patient visits to other hospitals

Service use by those living in residential accommodation

Twenty two percent of residents in all residential facilities had a GP consultation within the two weeks prior to interview. Half of them saw their GPs because of a physical complaint, about a third had a consultation for a mental health problem and the remainder said they contacted their GP for both physical and mental problems. Residents with schizophrenia living in hostels were most likely to consult their GP for a mental health problem, 17%, and least likely to see their GP for a physical complaint, 6%. Conversely, those living in supported housing or recognised lodgings were most likely to consult their GP for a physical complaint, 17%, and least likely to see their GP for a mental health problem, 9%. *(Table 1.19)*

Within the previous 12 months, the proportion of residents who had a GP consultation was 76%, with two thirds of them, 53%, seeking treatment or advice on a mental health problem. Again, adults with schizophrenia living in ordinary housing or recognised lodging were least likely to have seen their GPs in the past 12 months for a mental health problem: 4 in 10 had a GP consultation for a mental health problem compared with 5 in 10 of those in residential care homes and about 6 in 10 of group home or hostel residents. Characteristics which at least doubled the odds of a GP consultation in the past year were living in unsupervised accommodation, being a woman, and having a long-standing physical complaint. *(Tables 1.20 to 1.21)*

In-patient stays in hospital in the past 12 months were rare events. Five percent of residents had been in hospital because of a physical health problem and only one percent with a mental health problem. Out-patient visits, however, were made by 56% of residents including 43% who had a consultation or treatment for a mental health problem. Among the various residential facilities, the largest proportion of residents

who attended as out-patients for a mental health problem, 54%, was among those living in ordinary housing or recognised lodging. The characteristics which roughly doubled the odds of having any out-patient visit was being a woman, having some rather than no qualifications, and living in unsupervised accommodation. Two thirds of residents had their out-patient appointments in an out-patients department of a hospital, a quarter went to a clinic or Health Centre and an eighth went to a Day Centre for treatment. Nearly all attenders said they saw a psychiatrist or a psychiatric nurse and were currently attending hospitals, clinics or centres for out-patient treatment or check-ups.
(Tables 1.22 to 1.25)

Overall 8 in 10 residents with schizophrenia living in residential accommodation had at least one domiciliary visit in the past 12 months. Social workers saw the largest proportion of residents, 46%, closely followed by community psychiatric nurses, 39%. A fifth of residents had been visited by a home care worker and a sixth by a psychiatrist. The extent to which residents received domiciliary visits by homecare workers and psychiatrists showed the greatest variation by type of accommodation. Homecare workers tended predominantly to visit those in group homes and supported accommodation whereas psychiatrists were more in demand in hostels and residential care homes. The nature of the work carried out by the various professionals who made domiciliary visits is reflected in the frequency of their calls. Most home care workers visited their clients at least once a week, with a half seeing residents every day. Psychiatrists were called to see residents normally less than once a month. *(Tables 1.26 to 1.27)*

When asked whether they had turned down any domiciliary service in the past 12 months, 10% of residents said they had. The significance of this finding depends on which services were offered to how many people in the first place and this information was not collected in the survey. Taking this cautionary note into account, 40% of those who turned down any domiciliary service said they did not want to be seen by a social worker, 30% refused a visit by a psychiatrist, and 23% did not want a psychiatric nurse to call. (*Table 1.28*)

The same proportion of residents, 10% also reported that they sometimes decided not to see a doctor or other professional when they themselves or others around them thought they should. (*Table 1.29*)

Service use by hospital residents

Six percent of hospital residents had an in-patient stay at another hospital mostly for a physical complaint.

Twenty two percent of all hospital residents had out-patient appointments at other hospitals comprising 34% of private hospital, clinic or nursing home residents, 23% of patients in NHS psychiatric hospitals and 9% of those in

psychiatric units or wards of general hospitals. Because most out-patient stays were for physical complaints, these differences were most likely due to the availability of services at the residents' own hospital. General hospitals are far more likely to have the staff and facilities relevant to treating physical complaints than psychiatric hospitals or private nursing homes. (*Tables 1.30 to 1.31*)

Footnotes and references

1. See Appendix A for a general description of how the psychiatric morbidity of residents of institutions were arrived at. Full details of the methodology of the institutional survey are provided in Report 4 of this series of Reports.

2. Appendix A shows the diagnostic algorithms for translating responses to the CIS-R questionnaire into ICD-10 disorder categories.

Table 1.1 Personal characteristics of residents by sex

Residents with schizophrenia, delusional or schizoaffective disorders

	Men	Women	All
	%	%	%
Age			
16-24	4	7	5
25-34	24	13	20
35-44	24	21	23
45-54	28	30	29
55-64	20	30	23
Marital status			
Married/cohabiting	2	7	3
Single	86	66	80
Widowed	1	4	2
Divorced	10	21	13
Separated	2	3	2
Ethnicity			
White or European	90	95	91
West Indian or African	7	3	6
Asian or Oriental	3	2	2
Other	1	0	1
Qualifications			
A level or higher	10	10	10
GCSE/ O level	9	13	10
Other qualifications	8	7	8
No qualifications	72	70	72
Base	*586*	*242*	*828*
% of men and women with schizophrenia	71%	29%	100%

Table 1.2   Personal characteristics of residents by age and sex

Residents with schizophrenia, delusional or schizoaffective disorders

	Men					Women					All adults
	16-34	35-44	45-54	55-64	All men	16-34	35-44	45-54	55-64	All women	
	%	%	%	%	%	%	%	%	%	%	%
Marital status											
Married/cohabiting	1	1	3	3	2	5	5	5	11	7	3
Single	94	87	85	75	86	87	69	61	54	66	80
Widowed	2	1	0	2	1	-	0	5	8	4	2
Divorced	2	10	10	20	10	8	20	29	21	21	13
Separated	1	2	2	1	2	-	5	0	6	3	2
Ethnicity											
White or European	77	94	95	94	90	84	97	97	97	95	91
West Indian or African	14	4	4	4	7	12	-	-	3	3	6
Asian or Oriental	6	1	2	2	3	2	3	3	-	2	2
Other	4	0	-	-	1	2	-	-	-	0	1
Qualifications											
A level or higher	11	12	10	8	10	8	18	4	12	10	10
GCSE/O level	12	13	6	6	9	25	16	11	5	13	10
Other qualifications	12	8	5	5	8	13	8	5	4	7	8
No qualifications	64	67	78	81	72	53	58	80	79	70	72
Base	*162*	*144*	*164*	*116*	*586*	*47*	*50*	*73*	*72*	*242*	*828*

Table 1.3   Personal characteristics of residents by type of institution

Residents with schizophrenia, delusional or schizoaffective disorders

	Hospitals	Residential care homes	Group homes	Hostels	Ordinary housing/ Recognised lodging	All*
	%	%	%	%	%	%
Sex						
Men	71	66	83	68	64	71
Women	29	34	17	32	36	29
Age						
16-34	31	23	18	24	13	25
35-44	20	22	22	37	28	23
45-54	27	33	34	24	22	29
55-64	22	21	25	16	37	23
Marital status						
Married/cohabiting	4	2	3	-	8	3
Single	79	82	80	81	77	80
Widowed	2	2	1	2	2	2
Divorced	13	14	12	15	10	13
Separated	2	1	3	2	3	2
Ethnicity						
White or European	89	92	95	93	96	91
West Indian or African	6	5	5	5	2	6
Asian or Oriental	4	2	-	-	2	2
Other	2	-	-	2	-	1
Qualifications						
A level or higher	8	8	15	20	15	10
GCSE/O level	9	12	13	6	17	10
Other qualifications	6	8	8	7	10	8
No qualifications	77	72	64	68	59	72
Base	*359*	*193*	*113*	*73*	*71*	*828*

* Includes 19 residents living in another type of residential accommodation.

Table 1.4   Odds ratios of socio-demographic characteristics associated with adults residing in hospitals compared with residential accommodation

Residents with schizophrenia, delusional or schizoaffective disorders

Factor	Adjusted Odds Ratio	95% Confidence Intervals
Age		
55-64	1.00	....
45-64	0.94	(0.64-1.39)
35-44	0.87	(0.57-1.32)
16-34	1.74**	(1.16-2.61)
Qualifications		
A level	1.00	....
GCSE/O levels	1.23	(0.65-2.32)
Other qualifications	1.06	(0.53-2.14)
No qualifications	1.94**	(1.19-3.17)

Other factors entered in the model were sex, ethnicity and marital status.

*p<0.05 **p<0.01

Table 1.5   Residence characteristics of residents by type of institution

Residents with schizophrenia, delusional or schizoaffective disorders

	Hospitals clinics & nursing homes	Residential care homes	Group homes	Hostels	Ordinary housing/ Recognised lodging	All*
	%	%	%	%	%	%
Length of stay						
Less than 1 year	21	23	17	23	10	20
1 year < 2 years	14	20	9	16	14	15
2 years < 3 years	19	14	14	14	16	17
3 years < 4 years	6	12	18	8	17	10
4 years < 5 years	5	6	12	18	8	8
5 years < 6 years	4	4	8	1	8	5
6 years < 7 years	1	5	2	2	0	2
7 years < 8 years	2	5	9	6	2	4
8 years < 9 years	3	2	5	4	6	3
9 years < 10 years	2	3	-	3	8	2
10 years < 15 years	6	4	7	5	9	6
15 years < 20 years	4	2	-	-	2	2
20 years < 25 years	3	-	-	-	-	1
25 years < 30 years	3	-	-	-	-	2
30 years < 35 years	4	-	-	-	-	2
35 years < 40 years	1	-	-	-	-	1
40 years or more	1	-	-	-	-	1
Mean length of stay (years)	7.2	3.6	4.2	3.6	4.8	5.3
(Mean age)	(43)	(44)	(46)	(43)	(48)	(44)
Median length of stay (years)	2.5	2.5	3.5	2.5	3.5	2.5
(Median age)	(44)	(46)	(47)	(41)	(49)	(45)
Where subject was living before present institution						
Hospital, clinic or nursing home	38	44	31	33	47	39
Private household	45	30	27	26	21	35
Supported accommodation/ group home	5	4	20	14	27	10
Residential care home	1	17	16	20	3	9
Prison/ on remand	6	1	-	-	-	3
B&B/ Hotel/ Hostel	2	2	2	5	2	2
Sleeping rough	1	-	1	2	0	1
Other	1	1	2	-	-	1
Base	*359*	*193*	*113*	*73*	*71*	*828*

* Includes 19 residents living in another type of residential accommodation

Table 1.6 Neurotic disorders and significant neurotic symptoms (as measured by the CIS-R) of residents by type of institution

Residents with schizophrenia, delusional and schizoaffective disorders who answered the CIS-R

		Hospitals clinics & nursing homes	Residential care homes	Group homes	Hostels	Ordinary housing/ Recognised lodging	All*
		%	%	%	%	%	%
Number of neurotic disorders	0	52	58	54	46	66	55
	1	34	28	28	47	26	31
	2	9	10	14	5	6	10
	3	4	4	1	2	2	3
	4	0	-	1	-	-	0
Any neurotic disorder		**48**	**42**	**46**	**54**	**34**	**45**

Percentage with each neurotic disorder

	Hospitals clinics & nursing homes	Residential care homes	Group homes	Hostels	Ordinary housing/ Recognised lodging	All*
Type of neurotic disorder						
Generalised Anxiety Disorder	21	24	29	20	15	22
Mixed anxiety and depressive disorder	4	18	15	12	10	10
Depressive episode	11	7	10	8	2	8
Phobia	6	9	11	6	7	8
Obsessive-Compulsive Disorder	7	6	10	2	2	6
Panic	6	2	2	9	4	5

Percentage with each neurotic symptom

	Hospitals clinics & nursing homes	Residential care homes	Group homes	Hostels	Ordinary housing/ Recognised lodging	All*
Significant neurotic symptoms						
Fatigue	47	44	44	55	24	43
Sleep problems	36	35	51	20	31	36
Worry	33	34	43	34	28	34
Anxiety	32	32	39	28	20	32
Concentration/forgetfulness	30	32	30	29	17	28
Depression	28	22	26	26	8	24
Depressive ideas	25	28	27	27	13	24
Obsessions	22	22	25	11	25	20
Irritability	22	19	19	21	16	20
Compulsions	23	10	24	16	19	18
Phobia	12	21	16	12	16	16
Panic	21	15	15	10	11	16
Worry about physical health	17	17	20	12	10	16
Somatic symptoms	19	11	11	12	10	13
Base	*220*	*147*	*96*	*59*	*59*	*596*

* Includes 14 residents living in another type of residential accommodation.

Table 1.7   Percentage of residents with each long standing physical complaint by sex

Residents with schizophrenia, delusional or schizoaffective disorders

	Men	Women	All
	Percentage with each complaint		
Nervous system complaints	**6**	**6**	**6**
Epilepsy	3	4	3
Huntington's chorea	1	1	1
Brain damage from infection/ injury	1	1	1
Parkinson's disease	0	0	0
Other nervous system complaints	1	0	1
Musculo-skeletal complaints	**4**	**10**	**6**
Arthritis/ rheumatism/ fibrositis	1	4	2
Back and neck problems/ slipped disk	1	1	1
Other problems of bones/ muscles/ joints	2	6	3
Endocrine/ nutritional/ metabolic diseases and immunity disorders	**3**	**8**	**5**
Diabetes	3	4	3
Hyper- or hypo- thyroidism	0	4	1
Other complaints	0	1	1
Heart and circulatory system complaints	**4**	**5**	**4**
Cerebral haemorrhage	0	1	1
Heart attack/ angina	1	1	1
Hypertension	1	2	1
Other complaints	2	2	2
Digestive system complaints	**4**	**4**	**4**
Respiratory system complaints	**2**	**1**	**2**
Skin complaints	**2**	**2**	**2**
Genito-urinary system complaints	**0**	**2**	**1**
Eye complaints	**1**	**2**	**1**
Ear complaints	**1**	**0**	**1**
Neoplasms (and benign lumps or cysts)	**1**	**1**	**1**
Infectious and parasitic diseases	**0**	**0**	**0**
Blood disorders	**0**	**1**	**0**
Any physical complaint	**21**	**27**	**23**
Base	*586*	*242*	*828*

Table 1.8   Percentage of residents with long standing physical complaints by age and sex

Residents with schizophrenia, delusional or schizoaffective disorders

Physical complaint	Age				
	16-34	35-44	45-54	55-64	All
	Percentage with each complaint				
Women					
Musculo- skeletal complaints	15	5	4	18	10
Nervous system complaints	8	3	5	7	6
Endocrine disorders	6	10	8	6	8
Heart/ circulation complaints	-	-	1	15	5
Digestive system complaints	5	0	-	10	4
Skin complaints	-	-	1	4	2
Respiratory system complaints	0	4	-	0	1
Eye complaints	1	-	2	3	2
Genito- urinary system complaints	-	2	3	4	2
Ear complaints	-	0	1	-	0
Neoplasms (and benign lumps or cysts)	-	-	-	2	1
Infectious and parasitic diseases	-	-	-	1	0
Blood disorders	-	1	1	1	1
Any physical complaint	**25**	**21**	**22**	**38**	**27**
Base	*47*	*50*	*73*	*72*	*242*
Men					
Musculo- skeletal complaints	4	3	5	3	4
Nervous system complaints	5	6	6	5	6
Endocrine disorders	3	4	4	4	3
Heart/ circulation complaints	1	5	7	5	4
Digestive system complaints	3	5	4	5	4
Skin complaints	2	2	1	2	2
Respiratory system complaints	-	2	3	3	2
Eye complaints	-	-	2	1	1
Genito- urinary system complaints	-	0	0	1	0
Ear complaints	0	2	1	-	1
Neoplasms (and benign lumps or cysts)	0	-	2	-	1
Infectious and parasitic diseases	-	2	-	-	0
Blood disorders	-	0	-	-	0
Any physical complaint	**14**	**21**	**27**	**22**	**21**
Base	*162*	*144*	*164*	*116*	*586*

Table 1.9   Percentage of residents with long-standing physical complaints by age and type of institution

Residents with schizophrenia, delusional or schizoaffective disorders

	Age				
	16-34	35-44	45-54	55-64	All
	Percentage with a physical complaint				
NHS/ Trust/ Private hospitals and nursing homes	18	17	25	18	20
Residential care homes	8	31	25	38	25
Alternative forms of residential accommodation	22	19	26	35	25
All residents	**17**	**21**	**25**	**28**	23
Bases					
NHS/ Trust/ Private hospitals and nursing homes	*112*	*71*	*96*	*80*	*359*
Residential care homes	*45*	*43*	*64*	*41*	*193*
Alternative forms of residential accommodation	*52*	*80*	*77*	*67*	*276*
All residents	*210*	*194*	*237*	*188*	*828*

Table 1.10 Proportion of residents taking each type of CNS drug and having therapy or counselling by type of institution

Residents with schizophrenia, delusional or schizoaffective disorders

	Hospitals clinics & nursing homes	Residential care homes	Group homes	Hostels	Ordinary housing/ Recognised lodging	All*
	Percentage of adults using each type of drug					
Drugs used in psychoses and related conditions	98	90	91	91	94	94
Antipsychotic drugs	85	80	76	89	68	81
Depot injections	41	27	33	21	41	34
Antimanic drugs	8	13	9	17	10	11
Anticholinergic drugs	59	63	55	65	47	59
Anti- epileptics	15	9	7	14	6	12
Antidepressant drugs	12	20	19	19	10	16
Tricyclic antidepressants	7	16	18	15	10	12
Serotonin reuptake inhibitors	5	3	4	4	-	4
Hypnotics and anxiolytics	18	24	15	8	8	17
Hypnotics	15	19	10	8	8	14
Anxiolytics	5	8	4	-	1	5
Analgesics	8	2	4	5	1	5
Drugs used in nausea and vertigo	1	-	-	-	2	1
Drugs used in treatment of substance dependence	-	1	-	2	-	0
Any CNS Drugs	98	93	96	94	94	96
Any therapy or counselling	28	18	25	10	21	23
Base	*359*	*193*	*113*	*73*	*71*	*828*

* Includes 19 residents living in another type of residential accommodation.

15

Table 1.11 Proportion of residents taking each type of CNS drug and having counselling or therapy by presence of neurotic disorder (measured by CIS-R)

Residents with schizophrenia, delusional or schizoaffective disorders who answered the CIS-R
living in residential accommodation

	No neurotic disorder	With a neurotic disorder	All with a CIS-R interview
	Proportion of adults using each type of drug		
Drugs used in psychoses and related conditions	95	95	95
Antipsychotic drugs	82	86	84
Depot injections	36	34	35
Antimanic drugs	11	13	12
Anticholinergic drugs	59	59	59
Hypnotics and anxiolytics	12	21	16
Hypnotics	11	17	14
Anxiolytics	2	6	4
Antidepressant drugs	14	24	18
Tricyclic antidepressants	11	17	14
Serotonin reuptake inhibitors	4	7	5
Anti- epileptics	11	12	12
Analgesics	4	6	5
Drugs used in nausea and vertigo	1	1	1
Drugs used in substance dependence	1	1	1
Any CNS drugs	97	98	98
Any therapy or counselling	15	25	20
Base	*329*	*266*	*596*

Table 1.12 Percentage of residents who sometimes do not take their medication by personal and institution characteristics

Residents with schizophrenia, delusional or schizoaffective disorders who are being treated with antipsychotic drugs

	Percentage who do not take their drugs	Base
Sex		
Men	18	472
Women	14	201
Age		
16-34	29	178
35-44	15	159
45-54	10	195
55-64	12	141
Ethnicity		
White	16	614
Non- White	16	59
Qualifications		
A level or higher	32	70
GCSE/O level	19	76
Other qualifications	11	53
No qualifications	14	474
Physical complaint		
Has a physical complaint	19	151
No physical complaint	16	521
Length of stay		
Less than 1 year	24	140
1 year < 2 years	20	99
2 years < 3 years	12	107
3 years < 5 years	19	127
5 years or more	11	200
Type of institution		
Hospital, clinic or nursing home	16	305
Residential care home	10	154
Other residential accommodation	21	213
Degree of supervision		
Supervised	16	628
Unsupervised*	31	45
All residents	**16**	673

* Residents of unstaffed group homes and unsupervised ordinary housing or recognised lodging.

Table 1.13 Odds ratios of socio-demographic and institution characteristics associated with non-compliance with taking medication

Residents with schizophrenia, delusional or schizoaffective disorders who are being treated with antipsychotic drugs

Factor	Adjusted Odds Ratios#	95%CI
Age		
55-64	1.00	....
45-54	0.83	(0.41-1.68)
35-44	1.21	(0.61-2.41)
16-34	3.25**	(1.75-6.03)
Qualifications		
No qualifications	1.00	....
Other qualifications	0.48	(0.19-1.24)
GCSE O level	1.02	(0.53-1.97)
A level or higher	2.52**	(1.40-4.55)
Degree of supervision		
Supervised	1.00	....
Unsupervised##	2.54*	(1.24-5.21)

* p<0.05 **p<0.01

Residents of unstaffed group homes and unsupervised ordinary housing or recognised lodging.

\# Other factors entered in the model were sex, ethnicity, physical complaint, length of stay and type of institution.

Table 1.14   Last time antipsychotic drugs not taken and reason for abstention by age

Residents with schizophrenia, delusional or schizoaffective disorders who are being treated with antipsychotic drugs who sometimes had not taken their medication

	Age		
	16-34	35-64	All
	%	%	%
Last time antipsychotic drugs not taken			
Less than 1 week ago	53	48	50
At least 1 week ago but less than 1 month ago	17	18	18
At least 1 month ago	30	35	32
Reasons for not taking antipsychotic drugs			
Percentage giving each reason			
Did not like to take drugs	35	23	29
Forgot	15	38	28
Did not feel they were needed	13	15	13
Side effects	13	-	6
Other answers	30	31	31
Base	*51*	*60*	*111*

Table 1.15   Percentage of residents who sometimes take more of their medication by personal and institution characteristics

Residents with schizophrenia, delusional or schizoaffective disorders who are being treated with antipsychotic drugs

	Percentage who sometimes take more of their drugs	Base
Sex		
Men	5	472
Women	5	201
Age		
16-34	5	178
35-44	10	159
45-54	4	195
55-64	2	141
Ethnicity		
White	6	614
Non- White	2	59
Qualifications		
A level or higher	12	70
GCSE/O level	9	76
Other qualifications	8	53
No qualifications	3	474
Physical complaint		
Has a physical complaint	6	151
No physical complaint	3	521
Length of stay		
Less than 1 year	5	140
1 year < 2 years	5	99
2 years < 3 years	3	107
3 years < 5 years	6	127
5 years or more	6	200
Type of institution		
Hospital, clinic or nursing home	2	305
Residential care home	5	154
Other residential accommodation	11	213
Degree of supervision		
Supervised	4	628
Unsupervised*	23	45
All residents	5	673

* Residents of unstaffed group homes and unsupervised ordinary housing or recognised lodging

Table 1.16   Odds ratios of socio-demographic and institution characteristics associated with over-consumption of medication

Residents with schizophrenia, delusional or schizoaffective disorders who are being treated with antipsychotic drugs

Factor	Adjusted Odds Ratios##	95% CI
Age		
55-64	1.00	....
45-54	1.69	(0.43-6.70)
35-44	4.67*	(1.32-16.56)
16-34	2.65	(0.69-10.20)
Type of institution		
Hospital, clinic or nursing home	1.00	....
Residential care home	3.48*	(1.09-11.11)
Other residential accommodation	4.70**	(1.58-14.00)
Degree of supervision		
Supervised	1.00	....
Unsupervised#	3.85**	(1.52-9.73)

* p<0.05 **p<0.01

\#   Residents of unstaffed group homes and unsupervised ordinary
    housing or recognised lodging.
\#\# Other factors entered in the model were sex, ethnicity,
    qualifications, physical complaint and length of stay.

Table 1.17   Percentage of residents who had previously been given a different treatment for their condition by personal and institution characteristics

Residents with schizophrenia, delusional or schizoaffective disorders who are being treated with antipsychotic drugs

	Percentage who had been given a different treatment	*Base*
Sex		
Men	57	*472*
Women	55	*201*
Age		
16-34	65	*178*
35-44	54	*159*
45-54	55	*195*
55-64	51	*141*
Ethnicity		
White	56	*614*
Non- White	57	*59*
Qualifications		
A level or higher	67	*70*
GCSE/O level	61	*76*
Other qualifications	66	*53*
No qualifications	53	*474*
Physical complaint		
Has a physical complaint	57	*151*
No physical complaint	54	*521*
Length of stay		
Less than 1 year	54	*140*
1 year < 2 years	61	*99*
2 years < 3 years	58	*107*
3 years < 5 years	56	*127*
5 years or more	55	*200*
Type of institution		
Hospital, clinic or nursing home	63	*305*
Residential care home	46	*154*
Other residential accommodation	55	*213*
Degree of supervision		
Supervised	56	*628*
Unsupervised*	65	*45*
All residents**	**56**	*673*

*   Residents of unstaffed group homes and unsupervised ordinary
    housing or recognised lodging.
** 95% had stopped their previous treatment on professional
    advice.

Table 1.18 Percentage of residents who had refused alternative treatment or medication for their condition by personal and institution characteristics

Residents with schizophrenia, delusional or schizoaffective disorders who are being treated with antipsychotic drugs

	Percentage who refused a different treatment/medication	Base
Sex		
Men	12	472
Women	10	201
Age		
16-34	14	178
35-44	13	159
45-54	12	195
55-64	6	141
Ethnicity		
White	12	614
Non- White	3	59
Qualifications		
A level or higher	24	70
GCSE/O level	14	76
Other qualifications	12	53
No qualifications	9	474
Physical complaint		
Has a physical complaint	7	151
No physical complaint	12	521
Length of stay		
Less than 1 year	15	140
1 year < 2 years	12	99
2 years < 3 years	6	107
3 years < 5 years	12	127
5 years or more	10	200
Type of institution		
Hospital, clinic or nursing home	10	305
Residential care home	10	154
Other residential accommodation	14	213
Degree of supervision		
Supervised	11	628
Unsupervised*	16	45
All residents**	**11**	673

* Residents of unstaffed group homes and unsupervised ordinary housing or recognised lodging.

** Most residents had refused a different brand of antipsychotic drug or depot injections instead of oral medication.

Table 1.19   GP consultation in past two weeks by type of residential accommodation

Residents with schizophrenia, delusional or schizoaffective disorders living in residential accommodation

	Residential care homes	Group homes	Hostels	Ordinary housing or recognised lodging	All
	Percentage of residents in each facility having GP consultations				
Consulted GP in past two weeks for.....					
Physical and mental complaints	6	3	2	1	4
Mental health problem only	4	10	15	8	7
Physical health problem only	11	8	4	16	11
Any consultation	**21**	**20**	**21**	**25**	**22**
Base	*193*	*113*	*73*	*71*	*470*
Any consultation for a mental health problem	10%	13%	17%	9%	11%
Any consultation for a physical health problem	17%	11%	6%	17%	15%

Table 1.20   GP consultation in past twelve months by type of residential accommodation

Residents with schizophrenia, delusional or schizoaffective disorders living in residential accommodation

	Residential care homes	Group homes	Hostels	Ordinary housing or recognised lodging	All
	Percentage of residents in each facility having GP consultations				
Consulted GP in past 12 months for.....					
Physical and mental complaints	35	40	28	27	34
Mental health problem only	18	20	29	12	19
Physical health problem only	20	22	20	34	23
Any consultation	**73**	**82**	**77**	**74**	**76**
Base	*193*	*113*	*73*	*71*	*470*
Any consultation for a mental health problem	53%	60%	57%	39%	53%
Any consultation for a physical health problem	55%	62%	48%	61%	59%

Table 1.21 Odds ratios of socio-demographic and institution characteristics associated with having had a GP consultation in the past twelve months

Residents with schizophrenia, delusional or schizoaffective disorders living in residential accommodation

Factor	Adjusted Odds Ratios*	95% CI
Degree of supervision		
Supervised	1.00	....
Unsupervised	2.55*	(1.10-5.93)
Sex		
Male	1.00	....
Female	2.08**	(1.20-3.57)
Physical complaint		
No	1.00	....
Yes	1.98*	(1.12-3.50)
Qualifications		
No qualifications	1.00	....
Other qualifications	0.29***	(0.14-0.60)
GCSE/O level	0.96	(0.49-1.90)
A level or higher	1.19	(0.57-2.46)

* $p<0.05$ ** $p<0.01$ *** $p<0.001$

Other factors entered in the model were age, ethnicity, length of stay, type of accommodation.

Table 1.22   In-patient stays in past twelve months by type of residential accommodation

Residents with schizophrenia, delusional or schizoaffective disorders living in residential accommodation

	Residential care homes	Group homes	Hostels	Ordinary housing or recognised lodging	All
	Percentage of residents in each facility with an in-patient stay				
Had in-patient stay in past twelve months for.....					
Physical and mental complaints	1	2	-	-	1
Mental health problem only	-	-	-	-	-
Physical health problem only	7	3	3	2	4
Any in-patient stay	8	6	3	2	6
Base	*193*	*113*	*73*	*71*	*470*
Any in-patient stay for a mental health problem	1%	2%	-	-	1%
Any in-patient stay for a physical health problem	8%	5%	3%	2%	5%

Table 1.23   Out-patient visits in past twelve months by type of residential accommodation

Residents with schizophrenia, delusional or schizoaffective disorders living in residential accommodation

	Residential care homes	Group homes	Hostels	Ordinary housing or recognised lodging	All
	Percentage of residents in each facility with an out-patient visit				
Had out-patient visit in past twelve months for.....					
Physical and mental complaints	1	4	3	4	2
Mental health problem only	36	41	41	50	41
Physical health problem only	15	11	11	10	13
Any in-patient stay	52	56	55	60	56
Base	*193*	*113*	*73*	*71*	470
Any out-patient visit for a mental health problem	37%	45%	44%	54%	43%
Any out-patient visit for a physical health problem	16%	15%	14%	14%	15%

Table 1.24   Odds ratios of socio-demographic and institution characteristics associated with an out-patient visit in the past twelve months

Residents with schizophrenia, delusional or schizoaffective disorders living in residential accommodation

Factor	Adjusted Odds Ratio	95% Confidence Intervals
Degree of supervision		
Supervised	1.00	....
Unsupervised	2.20*	(1.17-4.14)
Sex		
Male	1.00	....
Female	2.10***	(1.36-3.23)
Qualifications		
No qualifications	1.00	....
Other qualifications	2.22	(1.05-4.67)
GCSE/O level	1.74	(0.93-3.24)
A level or higher	1.83	(1.00-3.35)

*p<0.05 **p<0.01
Other factors entered in the model were age, ethnicity, physical complaint, length of stay and type of institution.

Table 1.25   Characteristics of out-patient episodes for mental health problems

Residents with schizophrenia, delusional or schizoaffective disorders living in residential accommodation who had an out-patient visit in past twelve months for mental health problem

Where resident went to for treatment or check-up	*Percentage of residents* attending each place*
Out-patients department of hospital	68
Clinic or Health Centre	25
Day Centre	12
Other place	4
Who resident reported seeing at out-patient appointment	*Percentage of residents* seeing each professional*
Psychiatrist	78
Psychiatric nurse	34
Social worker/ counsellor	9
Other consultant/ hospital doctor	6
Occupational therapist	4
Psychologist	3
Other professional	6
Whether currently attending hospitals, clinics or centres for out-patient treatment or check-up	*Percentage of residents* currently attending*
Currently attending	95
Not currently attending	5
Base	*203*

* Percentages sum to more than 100% because some residents went to several places or saw several professionals

Table 1.26   Domiciliary visits in past twelve months by type of residential accommodation

Residents with schizophrenia, delusional or schizoaffective disorders living in residential accommodation

	Residential care homes	Group homes	Hostels	Ordinary housing or recognised lodging	All*
	Percentage of residents in each facility receiving the service				
Type of domiciliary visit in past twelve months					
Social worker	46	49	51	29	46
Community psychiatric nurse	40	42	34	45	39
Home Care worker	8	41	14	38	21
Psychiatrist	20	10	26	6	16
Voluntary worker	8	8	4	11	8
Occupational Therapist	8	6	6	4	6
Any domiciliary visit	**75**	**87**	**73**	**81**	**79**
Base	*193*	*113*	*73*	*71*	*470*

* Includes 19 residents in other sorts of residential accommodation.

Table 1.27   Frequency of and satisfaction with domiciliary visits

Residents with schizophrenia, delusional or schizoaffective disorders living in residential accommodation who have domiciliary visits

| | Type of domiciliary visit | | | | | |
	Social Worker	Community Psychiatric nurse	Home care worker	Psychiatrist	Voluntary work	Occupational Therapist
	%	%	%	%	%	%
Frequency of domiciliary visit						
4 or more times a week	6	3	51	-	10	[6]
2 or 3 times a week	6	7	18	-	4	[3]
Once a week	13	17	19	-	42	[7]
Less than once a week but at least once a month	27	41	9	4	20	[4]
Less than once a month	48	32	3	96	23	[8]
Degree of satisfaction with help or support provided						
Very satisfied	60	62	66	38	74	[16]
Fairly satisfied	28	27	30	50	26	[9]
Fairly dissatisfied	5	6	2	7	-	[2]
Very dissatisfied	7	6	2	5	-	[1]
Base	*216*	*184*	*95*	*76*	*35*	*28*

Table 1.28 Refusal of help or support in past twelve months

Residents with schizophrenia, delusional or schizoaffective disorders living in residential accommodation

Proportion of residents who turned down help or support in the past twelve months	10%	(Base=470)

Percentage of residents who turned down each type of help*

Type of help turned down was offered by.....

Social Worker	40
Psychiatrist	30
Community Psychiatric nurse	23
Occupational Therapist	14
Home help	11
Voluntary work	3
Other sources of help	8

Reason help turned down

Not wanted or needed	40
Didn't think it could help	34
Couldn't face it	18
Did not like people offering help	16
Other reasons	1
Base	*47*

*Percentages sum to more than 100% as some residents gave several answers to each question

Table 1.29 Not seeking medical help when others thought they should

Residents with schizophrenia, delusional or schizoaffective disorders living in residential accommodation

Proportion of residents who decided not to see a doctor or other professional when they themselves or others around them thought they should	10%	(Base=470)

Percentage of residents who gave each reason for not seeking help*

Did not think it was necessary	27
Thought problem would get better by itself	15
Afraid of consequences (hospitalisation, treatment)	13
Did not think anyone could help	10
Felt it was a problem they should be able to cope with	7
Didn't have the time	5
Afraid of side effects of treatment	3
Other answers	38
Base	*51*

* Percentages sum to more than 100% as some residents gave several reasons

Table 1.30   Services received at own hospital

Residents with schizophrenia, delusional schizoaffective disorders living in hospital

	NHS/Trust Psychiatric hospital	NHS/Trust Psychiatric unit or ward of General hospital	Private hospital, clinic or nursing home	All
	Percentage of residents receiving each service			
Who patient has seen in own hospital in past twelve months				
Psychiatrist	88	90	92	88
Other consultant or hospital doctor	31	23	22	29
Psychiatric nurse	89	99	88	90
Occupational Therapist	49	45	30	43
Social worker/counsellor	44	45	30	43
Psychologist	19	18	45	23
Voluntary worker	15	16	23	16
Base	*257*	*53*	*49*	*359*

Table 1.31   In-patient stays and out-patient visits to other hospitals

Residents with schizophrenia, delusional or schizoaffective disorders living in hospital

	NHS/Trust Psychiatric hospital	NHS/Trust Psychiatric unit or ward of General hospital	Private hospital, clinic or nursing home	All
Proportion of hospital residents with in-patient stays in other hospitals in past twelve months for.....				
Physical and mental health problem	1	-	-	0
Mental health problem only	-	-	-	-
Physical health problem only	6	5	3	5
Any in-patient stay in other hospital	**6**	**5**	**3**	**6**
Proportion of hospital residents who had out-patient visits to other hospitals in past twelve months for.....				
Physical and mental health problem	2	-	5	2
Mental health problem only	1	1	2	1
Physical health problem only	20	8	27	19
Any out-patient visit to other hospital	**23**	**9**	**34**	**22**
Base	*257*	*53*	*49*	*359*

2   Residents with affective psychoses

2.1   Introduction

Residents were classified as having an affective psychosis if they or staff, acting as proxy informants with the informed consent of residents, said they were suffering from mania or bipolar affective disorder. Residents were more likely to use the expressions such as manic depression or mood swings.

Ninety six residents, approximately 8% of the total sample, were identified as having one of these disorders. Because of this relatively small number, compared with residents who were identified as having schizophrenia, delusional or schizoaffective disorders, analysis by institutional type has been limited to examining differences in the characteristics of residents living in hospitals with those in all types of residential accommodation.

2.2   Descriptive profile of residents

Among residents with affective psychosis living in institutions, 56% were men, 65% were single, and 58% had no qualifications. Most strikingly, a quarter of all residents were divorced, double the proportion of those with schizophrenia. Hospital patients with affective psychosis tended to be younger and less well qualified than those living in residential facilities.

In all types of institution, the residents' mean length of stay was four years yet the median value was two and a half years. This difference was mainly due to the 20% of residents who had been in hospital for at least ten years. Residents with affective psychosis were similar to those with schizophrenia in that about fifty

percent who answered the CIS-R were ascribed a neurotic disorder. In both cases, General Anxiety Disorder was found to be the most prevalent disorder, affecting about a third of those with affective psychosis. *(Tables 2.1 to 2.4)*

2.2   Physical complaints

Forty two percent of residents with affective psychosis reported a long-standing physical complaint, predominantly disorders of the nervous system or problems with the musculo-skeletal system. A quarter of male residents with affective psychosis said they had epilepsy. This may be indicative of the epileptic symptoms which can result from taking certain types of antipsychotic medication. *(Tables 2.5 to 2.6)*

2.3   Treatment

The proportions of residents with affective psychosis taking each category of CNS drug were remarkably similar across types of institutions. About 8 in 10 were reported to be on drugs used in treating psychosis and related conditions with about half this group taking antimanic drugs. About 3 in 10 were taking antidepressants, roughly equal proportions taking tricyclic antidepressants and specific serotonin reuptake inhibitors. The fairly extensive use of anticholinergic drugs and antiepileptics, taken by 40% and 34% of residents respectively, most probably represents a widespread method of controlling side effects of the antipsychotic drugs. A third of residents were also undergoing some form of counselling or therapy. *(Table 2.7)*

The attitudes and behaviour of residents with affective psychosis with respect to their medication were very similar to those with schizophrenia: 17% sometimes did not take their drugs, 6% sometimes took more than the stated dose, 59% previously had a different treatment for their condition, and 13% had refused treatment in the past year. *(Table 2.8)*

2.4   Use of services

Among the 45 residents with affective psychosis living in residential accommodation, 27% had consulted their GP in the past 2 weeks and 78% in the past 12 months. Of those who had consulted their GP in the past year, a half had seen their GP for both mental and physical complaints, a quarter for a physical disorder and the remaining quarter for a mental health problem only.

One in seven of all occupants of residential accommodation had an in-patient stay in hospital in the 12 months prior to interview, mostly for a physical health problem. However, out-patient visits, made by 6 in 10 residents, were largely for treatment or check-ups relating to their mental disorder. Just over three-quarters of residents had a domiciliary visit in the past year and two thirds of those in receipt of any such service were seen by a social worker.

Residents with affective psychosis were also similar to those with schizophrenia in that 13% had turned down a service offered to them and 12% said they had decided not to seek professional help when they knew they should have done. (Data not shown) *(Tables 2.9 to 2.10)*

Among the 51 hospital residents with affective psychosis, 12% had an in-patient stay in another hospital and 27% had attended an out-patient department in other premises. In most cases, contact with other hospitals was for a physical health problem. *(Table 2.11)*

Table 2.1 Personal characteristics of residents by sex

Residents with affective psychoses

	Men	Women	All
	%	%	%
Age			
16-24	8	18	12
25-34	27	23	25
35-44	23	16	20
45-54	27	24	26
55-64	15	20	17
Marital status			
Married/cohabiting	1	9	4
Single	72	56	65
Widowed	-	6	2
Divorced	22	26	24
Separated	5	4	4
Ethnicity			
White or European	93	94	94
West Indian or African	2	0	1
Asian or Oriental	1	6	3
Other	4	-	3
Qualifications			
A levels or higher	13	7	11
GCSE/O levels	26	29	27
Other qualifications	8	-	4
No qualifications	53	64	58
Base	*56*	*41*	*96*
% of men and women with affective psychoses	58%	42%	100%

Table 2.2 Personal characteristics of residents by type of institution

Residents with affective psychoses

	Hospitals clinics & nursing homes	Residential accomm-odation	All
	%	%	%
Sex			
Men	60	56	58
Women	40	44	42
Age			
16-34	49	23	37
35-44	11	31	20
45-54	25	26	26
55-64	15	20	17
Marital status			
Married/cohabiting	3	6	4
Single	72	57	65
Widowed	1	4	2
Divorced	22	26	24
Separated	2	7	4
Ethnicity			
White or European	92	95	94
West Indian or African	2	-	1
Asian or Oriental	1	5	3
Other	5	-	3
Qualifications			
A level or higher	12	9	11
GCSE/O level	16	40	27
Other qualifications	7	2	4
No qualifications	64	50	58
Base	*51*	*45*	*96*

Table 2.3   Residence characteristics of residents by type of institution

Residents with affective psychoses

Length of stay	Hospitals clinics and nursing homes	Residential accom- modation	All
	%	%	%
Less than 1 year	35	30	32
1 year < 2 years	18	7	13
2 years < 3 years	10	24	17
3 years < 4 years	3	7	5
4 years < 5 years	7	4	6
5 years < 6 years	-	6	3
6 years < 7 years	1	15	7
7 years < 8 years	1	3	2
8 years < 9 years	3	2	2
9 years < 10 years	2	-	1
10 years < 15 years	12	1	6
15 years < 20 years	3	-	1
20 years < 25 years	5	-	2
Mean length of stay (years)	**4.7**	**3.1**	**4.0**
(Mean age)	**(38)**	**(43)**	**(41)**
Median length of stay (years)	**1.5**	**2.5**	**2.5**
(Median age)	**(35)**	**(42)**	**(38)**

Where subject was living before present institution			
Hospital, clinic or nursing home	36	45	40
Private household	47	24	36
Supported accommodation/ group home	3	15	8
Residential care home	7	10	8
Prison/ on remand	5	-	3
B&B/ Hotel/ Hostel	1	6	4
Other	1	-	1
Base	*51*	*45*	*96*

Table 2.4   Neurotic disorders and significant neurotic symptoms (as measured by the CIS-R) of residents

Residents with affective psychoses who answered the CIS-R

Number of neurotic disorders		%
	0	48
	1	22
	2	16
	3	12
	4	1
Any neurotic disorder		**52**

Type of neurotic disorder	
Generalised Anxiety Disorder	35
Depressive episode	22
Phobia	12
Obsessive-Compulsive Disorder	12
Mixed anxiety and depressive disorder	9
Panic	5

Significant neurotic symptoms	
Fatigue	49
Sleep problems	42
Anxiety	42
Worry	40
Depressive ideas	36
Depression	35
Concentration/forgetfulness	31
Irritability	24
Obsessions	22
Somatic symptoms	22
Worry about physical health	20
Compulsions	15
Phobia	13
Panic	12
Base	69

Table 2.5   Percentage of residents with each long standing physical complaint by sex

Residents with affective psychoses

	Men	Women	All
	Percentage with each complaint		
Nervous system complaints	29	9	21
Epilepsy	26	8	18
Brain damage from infection/ injury	3	2	3
Other nervous system complaints	1	0	1
Musculo-skeletal complaints	8	17	12
Arthritis/ rheumatism/ fibrositis	3	10	6
Back and neck problems/ slipped disk	1	2	1
Other problems of bones/ muscles/ joints	4	6	5
Endocrine/ nutritional/ metabolic dieases and immunity disorders	4	6	5
Diabetes	4	4	4
Hyper- or hypo- thyroidism	-	2	1
Heart and circulatory system complaints	5	4	5
Heart attack/ angina	3	-	2
Hypertension	-	2	1
Other complaints	4	2	3
Genito- urinary system complaints	1	10	5
Respiratory system complaints	1	9	4
Digestive system complaints	3	2	3
Eye complaints	6	0	3
Ear complaints	1	-	1
Skin complaints	-	2	1
Neoplasms (and benign lumps or cysts)	-	-	-
Infectious and parasitic diseases	-	-	-
Blood disorders	-	-	-
Any physical disorder	42	42	42
Base	*56*	*41*	*96*

Table 2.6   Percentage of residents with each long standing physical complaint by age

Residents with affective psychoses

	Age		All
	16-39	40-64	
	Percentage with each complaint		
Nervous system complaints	19	22	21
Epilepsy	18	19	18
Brain damage from infection/ injury	1	3	3
Other nervous system complaints	-	2	1
Musculo-skeletal complaints	14	10	12
Arthritis/ rheumatism/ fibrositis	2	9	6
Back and neck problems/ slipped disk	1	1	1
Other problems of bones/ muscles/ joints	10	-	5
Endocrine/ nutritional/ metabolic dieases and immunity disorders	3	6	5
Diabetes	3	5	4
Hyper- or hypo- thyroidism	-	2	1
Heart and circulatory system complaints	2	7	5
Heart attack/ angina	2	2	2
Hypertension	-	1	1
Other complaints	2	4	3
Genito- urinary system complaints	6	4	5
Respiratory system complaints	-	8	4
Digestive system complaints	2	3	3
Eye complaints	0	6	3
Ear complaints	-	1	1
Skin complaints	-	1	1
Neoplasms (and benign lumps or cysts)	-	-	-
Infectious and parasitic diseases	-	-	-
Blood disorders	-	-	-
Any physical disorder	40	44	42
Base	*48*	*48*	*96*

Table 2.7   Proportion of residents taking each type of CNS drug and having therapy or counselling by type of institution

Residents with affective psychoses

	Hospitals	All Residential accommodation	All
	Percentage of adults using each type of drug		
Drugs used in psychoses and related conditions	**76**	**83**	**79**
Antipsychotic drugs	66	60	63
Depot injections	21	22	22
Antimanic drugs	33	39	36
Anticholinergic drugs	**41**	**40**	**40**
Anti- epileptics	**41**	**26**	**34**
Antidepressant drugs	**27**	**29**	**28**
Tricyclic antidepressants	15	20	18
Serotonin reuptake inhibitors	16	8	13
Compound antidepressants	5	-	3
Hypnotics and anxiolytics	**26**	**19**	**23**
Hypnotics	20	15	18
Anxiolytics	11	4	8
Analgesics	**4**	**3**	**4**
Drugs used in nausea and vertigo	-	-	-
Drugs used in treatment of substance dependence	-	-	-
Any CNS drugs	**97**	**94**	**96**
Any therapy or counselling	**41**	**28**	**35**
Base	*51*	*46*	96

Table 2.8 Behaviour and attitudes on taking medication

Residents with affective psychoses taking any CNS drug

	%
Proportion of residents who sometimes did not take their medication even though they knew that they should	17
Proportion of residents who sometimes took more medication than the stated dose	6
Proportion of residents who have had other medication/ treatment for their condition*	59
Proportion of residents who had been offered any other medication or treatment for their condition which they turned down**	13
Base	92

* Five sixths of those who had other medication or treatment stopped on medical advice

** Proportion based on all residents on CNS drugs; number of residents offered other medication or treatment not known.

Table 2.9 Use of services

Residents with affective psychoses living in residential accommodation

	Consulted GP in past two weeks for.....	Consulted GP in past twelve months for.....	Had in-patient stay in past twelve months for.....	Had out-patient visit in past twelve months for.....
	%	%	%	%
Physical and mental complaints	3	41	4	-
Mental health problem only	15	18	-	48
Physical health problem only	8	19	10	10
Any consultation/ stay/ visit	**27**	**78**	**14**	**58**
Base	45	45	45	45
Any consultation/ stay/ visit for a mental health problem	18%	59%	4%	48%
Any consultation/ stay/ visit for a physical health problem	11%	60%	14%	10%

Table 2.10 Domiciliary visits in past twelve months

Residents with affective psychoses living in residential accommodation

	Percentage of residents in each facility receiving the service
Type of domiciliary visit in past twelve months	
Social worker	50
Community psychiatric nurse	28
Voluntary worker	17
Home Care worker	15
Psychiatrist	12
Occupational Therapist	9
Secondary voluntary worker	3
Any domiciliary visit	**78**
Base	*45*

Table 2.11 In-patient stays and out-patient visits to other hospitals

Residents with affective psychoses living in hospital

Proportion of hospital residents with in-patient stays in other hospitals in past twelve months for.....	
Physical and mental health problem	5
Mental health problem only	-
Physical health problem only	7
Any in-patient stay in other hospital	**12**
Proportion of hospital residents who had out-patient visits to other hospitals in past twelve months for.....	
Physical and mental health problem	1
Mental health problem only	4
Physical health problem only	22
Any out-patient visit to other hospital	**27**
Base	*51*

3   Residents with neurotic disorders

3.1   Introduction

One hundred and one residents, about 8% of the institutional sample, were identified as having a neurotic disorder, over three-quarters of them living in some type of residential accommodation. This group of residents, like all others in the survey, were asked to say what was the matter with them. Because they did not say anything indicative of schizophrenia or affective psychosis, their ascribed diagnosis was based on the CIS-R interview. However, a third of these residents, mostly living in group homes and recognised lodgings, reported taking antipsychotic drugs. This suggests that this particular group of residents, despite their medical history, felt they no longer considered themselves to have a psychotic illness. Living in residential accommodation rather than a hospital meant that this group of residents were more likely to have felt that they had got over their psychotic illness and were in the process of reintegrating themselves into the community. Therefore, the sample of residents described in this chapter is most likely a mixed group of residents: some genuinely having neurotic disorders and others who had psychotic disorders but still have significant neurotic symptoms.

3.2   Descriptive profile of residents

The biographical characteristics of residents with neurotic disorders were very similar to others living in institutions: their mean age was 40 and about two-thirds had never been married. However, those with neurotic disorders tended to be slightly better qualified with half of them having some educational qualifications and 1 in 5 having reached at least A-level standard.

The most marked difference between residents with neurotic disorders and those with other psychiatric complaints was that the mean length of stay of the neurotic group was 2.2 years compared with 5.3 years for those with schizophrenia. Nearly a half of all residents with neurosis had entered their present accommodation from private households. This suggests that some always had a neurotic disorder and were not adults who had recovered from a psychotic illness. *(Table 3.1 to 3.2)*

The distribution of the number of neurotic disorders showed that 68% of residents had one disorder, 19% had two, and 12% had three or more. More specifically, half the sample had Generalised Anxiety Disorder, just over a quarter had phobia or mixed anxiety and depressive disorder. Depressive episode and Obsessive-Compulsive Disorder was also present in about a fifth of cases. (Tables *3.3*)

3.3   Physical complaints

Half of all adults with neurotic disorders said they had a long-standing physical complaint. Musculo-skeletal problems, affecting 1 in 5 of residents, were most commonly reported, predominantly arthritis and rheumatism among women and those aged 40 or over. Respiratory and nervous system complaints mentioned by 12% and 8% of all residents who had neurotic disorders were more likely to be found among women aged under 40. Only men aged 40 or over mentioned any endocrine disorder and this was invariably diabetes. Compared with residents with affective psychoses, those with neuroses were far less likely to say they suffered from epilepsy: 1% compared with 18%. *(Tables 3.4 to 3.5)*

3.4   Treatment

Not surprisingly, the treatment regimes from those with neurosis was completely different than that for residents with schizophrenia or affective disorders. First, only two-thirds rather than all residents were on any CNS drugs, and second, antidepressants rather than antipsychotic drugs were the most commonly reported drugs taken by those who had a neurotic disorder. Hypnotic and anxiolytic drugs were also taken by a fifth of residents with neuroses. *(Table 3.6)*

The attitudes and behaviour of residents with neurotic disorders with respect to their medication was also very different from those with schizophrenia or affective psychosis. Forty five percent of the neurotic group sometimes did not take their drugs, and twenty one percent sometimes took more than the stated dose. This can be explained by the fact that those with neurotic disorders mostly lived in residential accommodation rather than hospitals. Among all residents, living in residential facilities, especially unstaffed accommodation, increased the odds of non-compliance. *(Table 3.7)*

3.5   Use of services

Among all groups living in residential accommodation, those with neurotic disorders were the most extensive users of primary care services: 34% had seen their GP in the past 2 weeks and 84% had consulted their GP in the past 12 months. Despite this degree of GP contact 1 in 5 residents said they sometimes did not seek professional help when they themselves or others around them thought they should.

However, residents with neurotic disorders were not very different from other groups in the proportions having in-patient stays, 13%, out-patient visits, 59%, or domiciliary visits from social workers, 42%. *(Tables 3.8 to 3.9)*

Table 3.1 Personal characteristics of residents by sex

Residents with neurotic disorders

	Men	Women	All
	%	%	%
Age			
16-24	14	33	21
25-34	16	21	18
35-44	22	20	21
45-54	23	14	20
55-64	26	12	20
Marital status			
Married/cohabiting	9	17	12
Single	66	64	65
Widowed	2	-	1
Divorced	18	19	19
Separated	5	-	3
Ethnicity			
White or European	96	89	93
West Indian or African	4	-	2
Asian or Oriental	1	7	3
Other	-	4	2
Qualifications			
A level or higher	12	27	18
GCSE/O level	24	6	17
Other qualifications	14	13	14
No qualifications	50	54	51
Base	*62*	*39*	*101*
% of men and women with neurotic disorders	61%	39%	100%

Table 3.2 Residence characteristics of residents by type of accommodation

Residents with neurotic disorders

	%
Length of stay	
Less than 1 year	39
1 year < 2 years	18
2 years < 3 years	16
3 years < 4 years	11
4 years < 5 years	5
5 years < 6 years	6
6 years < 7 years	3
7 years < 8 years	-
8 years < 9 years	2
9 years < 10 years	-
10 years < 15 years	1
Mean length of stay (years)	**2.2**
(Mean age)	**(40)**
Median length of stay (years)	**1.5**
(Median age)	**(40)**
Where subject was living before present institution	
Private household	46
Hospital, clinic or nursing home	21
Residential care home	13
B&B/ Hotel/ Hostel	10
Supported accommodation/ group home	7
Prison/ on remand	2
Base	*101*

Table 3.3 Neurotic disorders and significant neurotic symptoms (as measured by the CIS-R) of residents

Residents with neurotic disorders who answered the CIS-R

	%
Number of neurotic disorders	
1	68
2	19
3	9
4	3

	Percentage of adults with each neurotic disorder
Type of neurotic disorder	
Generalised Anxiety Disorder	47
Mixed anxiety and depressive disorder	27
Phobia	26
Depressive episode	20
Obsessive-Compulsive Disorder	19
Panic	7

	Percentage of adults with each neurotic sympton
Significant neurotic symptoms	
Depressive ideas	68
Worry	63
Sleep problems	59
Anxiety	59
Fatigue	56
Depression	56
Irritability	46
Obsessions	43
Concentration/forgetfulness	42
Phobia	39
Worry about physical health	34
Compulsions	29
Somatic symptoms	28
Panic	23
Base	*101*

Table 3.4 Percentage of residents with each long standing physical complaint by sex

Residents with neurotic disorders

	Men	Women	All
	Percentage with each complaint		
Musculo-skeletal complaints	12	29	19
Arthritis/ rheumatism/ fibrositis	8	22	14
Back and neck problems/ slipped disk	5	7	6
Other problems of bones/ muscles/ joints	2	-	1
Respiratory system complaints	6	22	12
Nervous system complaints	2	18	8
Epilepsy	2	-	1
Huntington's chorea	-	6	2
Migraine/ headaches	-	5	2
Other nervous system complaints	-	6	2
Digestive system complaints	7	9	8
Endocrine/ nutritional/ metabolic diseases and immunity disorders	11	-	7
Diabetes	11	-	7
Heart and circulatory system complaints	6	4	5
Heart attack/ angina	1	-	1
Hypertension	2	4	3
Other complaints	2	-	2
Ear complaints	-	7	3
Genito-urinary system complaints	-	5	2
Skin complaints	2	-	1
Blood disorders	-	4	1
Eye complaints	-	-	-
Neoplasms (and benign lumps or cysts)	-	-	-
Infectious and parasitic diseases	-	-	-
Any physical disorder	44	58	50
Base	*62*	*39*	*101*

43

Table 3.5 Percentage of residents with each long standing physical complaint by age

Residents with neurotic disorders

	16-39	40-64	All
	Percentage with each complaint		
Musculo-skeletal complaints	12	25	19
Arthritis/ rheumatism/ fibrositis	5	23	14
Back and neck problems/ slipped disk	5	6	6
Other problems of bones/ muscles/ joints	2	-	1
Respiratory system complaints	18	6	12
Nervous system complaints	12	4	8
Epilepsy	2	-	1
Huntington's chorea	5	-	2
Migraine/ headaches	0	4	2
Other nervous system complaints	5	-	2
Digestive system complaints	5	11	8
Endocrine/ nutritional/ metabolic diseases and immunity disorders	-	14	7
Diabetes	-	14	7
Heart and circulatory system complaints	-	10	5
Heart attack/ angina	-	1	1
Hypertension	-	6	3
Other complaints	-	3	2
Ear complaints	5	-	3
Genito- urinary system complaints	-	4	2
Skin complaints	2	-	1
Blood disorders	-	3	1
Eye complaints	1	2	-
Neoplasms (and benign lumps or cysts)	-	-	-
Infectious and parasitic diseases	-	-	-
Any physical disorder	42	57	50
Base	*51*	*50*	*101*

Table 3.6 Proportion of residents taking each type of CNS drug and having therapy or counselling

Residents with neurotic disorders

	Percentage of adults using each type of drug
Antidepressant drugs	44
Tricyclic antidepressants	28
Serotonin reuptake inhibitors	17
Monoamine oxidate inhibitors	2
Drugs used in psychoses and related conditions	35
Antipsychotic drugs	32
Depot injections	5
Antimanic drugs	4
Hypnotics and anxiolytics	21
Hypnotics	14
Anxiolytics	7
Analgesics	15
Anticholinergic drugs	12
Anti- epileptics	9
Drugs used in substance dependence	0
Any CNS Drugs	68
Any therapy or counselling	29
Base	*101*

Table 3.7 Behaviour and attitudes on taking medication

Residents with neurotic disorders taking any CNS drugs

	%
Proportion of residents who sometimes did not take their medication even though they knew that they should	45
Proportion of residents who sometimes took more medication than the stated dose	21
Proportion of residents who have had other medication/ treatment for their condition*	63
Proportion of residents who had been offered any other medication or treatment for their condition which they turned down**	12
Base	68

* Five sixths of those who had other medication or treatment stopped on medical advice

** Proportion based on all residents on CNS drugs; number of residents offered other medication or treatment not known.

Table 3.8 Use of services

Residents with neurotic disorders living in residential accommodation

	Consulted GP in past two weeks for.....	Consulted GP in past twelve months for.....	Had in-patient stay in past twelve months for.....	Had out-patient visit in past twelve months for.....
	%	%	%	%
Physical and mental complaints	-	44	3	-
Mental health problem only	13	10	-	31
Physical health problem only	21	30	10	28
Any consultation/ stay/visit	**34**	**84**	**13**	**59**
Base	*81*	*81*	*81*	*81*
Any consultation/ stay/ visit for a mental health problem	13%	54%	3%	31%
Any consultation/ stay/ visit for a physical health problem	21%	74%	13%	28%

Table 3.9 Domiciliary visits in past twelve months

Residents with neurotic disorders living in residential accommodation

Type of domiciliary visit in past twelve months	*Percentage of residents receiving the service*
Social worker	42
Community psychiatric nurse	18
Home Care worker	8
Psychiatrist	7
Occupational Therapist	7
Voluntary worker	3
Any domiciliary visit	**62**
Base	*81*

Appendix A Measuring psychiatric morbidity

A.1 Calculation of CIS-R symptom scores

Fatigue

Scores relate to fatigue or feeling tired or lacking in energy in the past week.

Score one for each of:
- Symptom present on four days or more
- Symptom present for more than three hours in total on any day
- Subject had to push him/herself to get things done on at least one occasion
- Symptom present when subject doing things he/she enjoys or used to enjoy at least once

Sleep problems

Scores relate to problems with getting to sleep, or otherwise, with sleeping more than is usual for the subject in the past week.

Score one for each of:
- Had problems with sleep for four nights or more
- Spent at least 1 hour trying to get to sleep on the night with least sleep
- Spent at least 1 hour trying to get to sleep on the night with least sleep
- Spent 3 hours or more truing to get to sleep on four nights or more
- Slept for at least 1 hour longer than usual for subject on any night
- Slept for at least 1 hour longer than usual for subject on any night
- Slept for more than 3 hours longer than usual for subject on four nights or more

Irritability

Scores relate to feelings of irritability, being short-tempered or angry in the past week.

Score one for each of:
- Symptom present for four days or more
- Symptom present for more than 1 hour on any day
- Wanted to shout at someone in past week (even if subject had not actually shouted)
- Had arguments, rows or quarrels or lost temper with someone and felt it was unjustified on at least one occasion

Worry

Scores relate to subject's experience of worry in the past week, other than worry about physical Health.

Score one for each of:
- Symptom present on 4 or more days
- Has been worrying too much in view of circumstances
- Symptom has been very unpleasant
- Symptom lasted over three hours in total on any day

Depression

Applies to subjects who felt sad, miserable or depressed or unable to enjoy or take an interest in things as much as usual, in the past week. Scores relate to the subject's experience in the past week.

Score one for each of:
- Unable to enjoy or take an interest in things as much as usual
- Symptom present on four days or more
- Symptom lasted for more than 3 hours in total on any day
- When sad, miserable or depressed subject did not become happier when something nice happened, or when in company

Depressive ideas

Applies to subjects who had a score of 1 for depression. Scores relate to experience in the past week.

Score one for each of:
- Felt guilty or blamed him/herself when things went wrong when it had not been his/her fault
- Felt not as good as other people
- Felt hopeless
- Felt that life isn't worth living
- Thought of killing him/herself

Anxiety

Scores relate to feeling generally anxious, nervous or tense in the past week. These feelings were not the result of a phobia.

Score one for each of:
- Symptom present on four or more days
- Symptom had been very unpleasant
- When anxious, nervous or tense, had one or more of following symptoms:
    heart racing or pounding
    hands sweating or shaking
    feeling dizzy
    difficulty getting breath
    butterflies in stomach
    dry mouth
    nausea or feeling as though he/she wanted to vomit

- Symptom present for more than three hours in total on any one day

Obsessions

Scores relate to the subject's experience of having repetitive unpleasant thoughts or ideas in the past week.

Score one for each of:

- Symptom present on four or more days
- Tried to stop thinking any of these thoughts
- Became upset or annoyed when had these thoughts
- Longest episode of the symptom was $1/4$ hour or longer

Concentration and forgetfulness

Scores relate to the subject's experience of concentration problems and forgetfulness in the past week.

Score one for each of:

- Symptoms present for four days or more
- Could not always concentrate on a TV programme, read a newspaper article or talk to someone without mind wandering
- Problems with concentration stopped subject from getting on with things he/she used to do or would have liked to do
- Forgot something important

Somatic symptoms

Scores relate to the subject's experience in the past week of any ache, pain or discomfort which was brought on or made worse by feeling low, anxious or stressed.

Score one for each of:

- Symptom present for four days or more
- Symptom lasted more than 3 hours on any day
- Symptom had been very unpleasant
- Symptom bothered subject when doing something interesting

Compulsions

Scores relate to the subject's experience of doing things over again when subject had already done them in the past week.

Score one for each of:

- Symptom present on four days or more
- Subject tried to stop repeating behaviour
- Symptom made subject upset or annoyed with him/herself
- Repeated behaviour three or more times when it had already been done

Phobias

Scores relate to subject's experience of phobias or avoidance in the past week

Score one for each of:

- Felt nervous/anxious about a situation or thing four or more times
- On occasions when felt anxious, nervous or tense, had one or more of following symptoms:
  heart racing or pounding
  hands sweating or shaking
  feeling dizzy
  difficulty getting breath
  butterflies in stomach
  dry mouth
  nausea or feeling as though he/she wanted to vomit
- Avoided situation or thing at least once because it would have made subject anxious, nervous or tense

Worry about physical health

Scores relate to experience of the symptom in the past week.

Score one for each of:

- Symptom present on four days or more
- Subject felt he/she had been worrying too much in view of actual health
- Symptom had been very unpleasant
- Subject could not be distracted by doing something else

Panic

Applies to subjects who felt anxious, nervous or tense in the past week and the scores relate to the resultant feelings of panic, or of collapsing and losing control in the past week.

Score one for each of:

- Symptom experienced once
- Symptom experienced more than once
- Symptom had been very unpleasant or unbearable
- An episode lasted longer than 10 minutes

A.2 Algorithms to produce ICD-10 psychiatric disorders

The mental disorders reported in Chapter 6 were produced from the CIS-R schedule which is described in Chapter 2 and reproduced in Appendix C. The production of the 6 categories of disorder shown in these tables occurred in 3 stages: first, the informants' responses to the CIS-R were used to produce specific ICD-10 diagnoses of neurosis.

This was done by applying the algorithms described below. Second, these specific neurotic disorders plus psychosis were arranged hierarchically and the 'highest' disorder assumed precedence. The actual precedence rules are described below. Finally, the range of ICD-10 diagnoses were grouped together to produce categories used in the calculation of prevalence.

It should be noted that as a result of the hierarchical coding described above, the diagnoses of the 6 neurotic disorders and the category of functional psychosis are exclusive: an individual included in the prevalence rates for one neurotic or psychotic disorder is not included in calculation of the rate for any other neurotic or psychotic disorder.

Algorithms for production of ICD-10 diagnoses of neurosis from the CIS-R ('scores' refer to CIS-R scores)

F32.00 Mild depressive episode without somatic symptoms

1. Symptom duration ≥ 2 weeks

2. *Two or more from:*

   - depressed mood
   - loss of interest
   - fatigue

3. *Two or three from:*

   - reduced concentration
   - reduced self-esteem
   - ideas of guilt
   - pessimism about future
   - suicidal ideas or acts
   - disturbed sleep
   - diminished appetite

4. Social impairment

5. *Fewer than four from:*

   - lack of normal pleasure /interest
   - loss of normal emotional reactivity
   - a.m. waking ≥ 2 hours early
   - loss of libido
   - diurnal variation in mood
   - diminished appetite
   - loss of ≥ 5% body weight
   - psychomotor agitation
   - psychomotor retardation

F32.01 Mild depressive episode with somatic symptoms

1. Symptom duration ≥ 2 weeks

2. *Two or more from:*

   - depressed mood
   - loss of interest
   - fatigue

3. *Two or three from:*

   - reduced concentration
   - reduced self-esteem
   - ideas of guilt
   - pessimism about future
   - suicidal ideas or acts
   - disturbed sleep
   - diminished appetite

4. Social impairment

5. *Four or more from:*

   - lack of normal pleasure /interest
   - loss of normal emotional reactivity
   - a.m. waking ≥ 2 hours early
   - loss of libido
   - diurnal variation in mood
   - diminished appetite
   - loss of 5% body weight
   - psychomotor agitation
   - psychomotor retardation

F32.10 Moderate depressive episode without somatic symptoms

1. Symptom duration ≥2 weeks

2. *Two or more* from:

   - depressed mood
   - loss of interest
   - fatigue

3. *Four or more* from:

   - reduced concentration
   - reduced self-esteem
   - ideas of guilt
   - pessimism about future
   - suicidal ideas or acts
   - disturbed sleep
   - diminished appetite

4. Social impairment

5. *Fewer than four* from:

   - lack of normal pleasure/interest
   - loss of normal emotional reactivity
   - a.m. waking ≥ 2 hours early
   - loss of libido
   - diurnal variation in mood
   - diminished appetite
   - loss of ≥ 5% body weight
   - psychomotor agitation
   - psychomotor retardation

F32.11 Moderate depressive episode with somatic symptoms

1. Symptom duration ≥2 weeks

2. *Two or more* from:

   - depressed mood
   - loss of interest
   - fatigue

3. *Four or more* from:

   - reduced concentration
   - reduced self-esteem
   - ideas of guilt
   - pessimism about future
   - suicidal ideas or acts
   - disturbed sleep
   - diminished appetite

4. Social impairment

5. *Four or more* from:

   - lack of normal pleasure /interest
   - loss of normal emotional reactivity
   - a.m. waking ≥2 hours early
   - loss of libido
   - diurnal variation in mood
   - diminished appetite
   - loss of ≥ 5% body weight
   - psychomotor agitation
   - psychomotor retardation

F32.2 Severe depressive episode

1. *All three* from:

   - depressed mood
   - loss of interest
   - fatigue

2. *Four or more* from:

   - reduced concentration
   - reduced self-esteem
   - ideas of guilt
   - pessimism about future
   - suicidal ideas or acts
   - disturbed sleep
   - diminished appetite

3. Social impairment

4. *Four or more* from:

   - lack of normal pleasure /interest
   - loss of normal emotional reactivity
   - a.m. waking ≥ 2 hours early
   - loss of libido
   - diurnal variation in mood
   - diminished appetite
   - loss of ≥ 5% body weight
   - psychomotor agitation
   - psychomotor retardation

F40.00 Agoraphobia without panic disorder

1. Fear of open spaces and related aspects: crowds, distance from home, travelling alone
2. Social impairment
3. Avoidant behaviour must be prominent feature
4. Overall phobia score ≥ 2
5. No panic attacks

F40.01 Agoraphobia with panic disorder

1. Fear of open spaces and related aspects: crowds, distance from home, travelling alone
2. Social impairment
3. Avoidant behaviour must be prominent feature
4. Overall phobia score ≥ 2
5. Panic disorder (overall panic score ≥ 2)

F40.1 Social phobias

1. Fear of scrutiny by other people: eating or speaking in public etc.
2. Social impairment
3. Avoidant behaviour must be prominent feature
4. Overall phobia score ≥ 2

F40.2 Specific (isolated) phobias

1. Fear of specific situations or things, e.g. animals, insects, heights, blood, flying, etc.
2. Social impairment
3. Avoidant behaviour must be prominent feature
4. Overall phobia score ≥ 2

F41.0 Panic disorder

1. Criteria for phobic disorders not met
2. Recent panic attacks
3. Anxiety-free between attacks
4. Overall panic score ≥ 2

F41.1 Generalised Anxiety Disorder

1. Duration ≥ 6 months
2. Free-floating anxiety
3. Autonomic overactivity
4. Overall anxiety score ≥ 2

F41.2 Mixed anxiety and depressive disorder

1. (Sum of scores for each CIS-R section) ≥ 12
2. Criteria for other categories not met

F42 Obsessive-Compulsive Disorder

1. Duration ≥ 2 weeks
2. At least one act/thought resisted
3. Social impairment
4. Overall scores:
   obsession score=4, or
   compulsion score=4, or
   obsession+compulsion scores ≥ 6

Hierarchical organisation of psychiatric disorders

The following rules (see table below) were used to allocate individuals who received more than one diagnosis of neurosis to the appropriate category.

Grouping neurotic and psychotic disorders into broad categories

The final step was to group some of the diagnoses into broad diagnostic categories prior to analysis.

Depressive episode

F32.00 and F32.01 were grouped to produce mild depressive episode (i.e. with or without somatic symptoms). F32.10 and F32.11 were similarly grouped to produce moderate depressive episode. Mild depressive episode, moderate depressive episode and Severe depressive episode (F32.2) were then combined to produce the final category of depressive episode.

Phobias

The ICD-10 phobic diagnoses F40.00, F40.01, F40.1 and F40.2, were combined into one category of phobia.

This produced six categories of neurosis for analysis:

Mixed anxiety and depressive disorder
Generalised Anxiety Disorder
Depressive episode
All phobias
Obsessive Compulsive Disorder
Panic disorder

Disorder 1	Disorder 2	Priority
Depressive episode (any severity)	Phobia	Depressive episode (any severity)
Depressive episode (mild)	OCD	OCD
Depressive episode (moderate)	OCD	Depressive episode (moderate)
Depressive episode (severe)	OCD	Depressive episode (severe)
Depressive episode (mild)	Panic disorder	Panic disorder
Depressive episode (moderate)	Panic disorder	Depressive episode (moderate)
Depressive episode (any severity)	GAD	Depressive episode (any severity)
Phobia (any)	OCD	OCD
Agoraphobia	GAD	Agoraphobia
Social phobia	GAD	Social phobia
Specific phobia	GAD	GAD
Panic disorder	OCD	Panic disorder
OCD	GAD	OCD
Panic disorder	GAD	Panic disorder

GAD = Generalised Anxiety Disorder; OCD = Obsessive– Compulsive Disorder

A3 Non-neurotic disorders

All psychiatric disorders with the exception of neuroses were assessed from self-reports by patients or their staff. Sometimes residents did not use medical terms to describe their conditions: how their answers were interpreted into ICD-10 diagnostic categories is shown below:

Primary diagnosis (based on ICD-10)

F00 - F09   Organic Mental Disorders
    Dementia
    Alzheimer's Disease

F10 - F19   Mental and behavioural disorders due to psychoactive substance use
    Alcohol/heavy drinker
    Opium
    Cannabis
    Sedatives
    Cocaine
    Stimulants
    Hallucinogens
    Tobacco
    Volatile solvents
    Any mixture of above

F20 - F29   Schizophrenia, schizotypal and delusional disorders
    Catatonic schizophrenia
    Chronic schizophrenia
    Hebephrenic schizophrenia
    High schizophrenia
    Mild schizophrenia
    Paranoid schizophrenia
    Schizophrenia
    Simple schizophrenia

    Auditory hallucinations
    Hallucinations
    Hearing voices
    Mild psychosis
    Psychosis
    Psychotic tendencies
    Schizo-affective disorder
    Schizophrenic affective disorder
    Voices

F30 - F39   Mood (affective) disorders (excluding depressive episode)
    Mania
    Hyperactive
    Hypomania
    Mania
    Manic depressive disorder
    Bipolar affective disorder
    Manic depression
    Manic depressive psychosis
    Moods
    Mood swings

F50 - F59   Behavioural syndromes associated with physiological disturbance and physical factors
    Anorexia nervosa
    Bulimia nervosa
    Sleep disorders (non-organic), nightfrights
    Sexual disorders (non-organic)
    Other behavioural syndromes

F60 - F69   Disorders of adult personality and behaviour
    Habit and impulse disorders
    Gender identity problems
    Other personality disorders

F70 - F79   Mental retardation
    Mental handicap
    Backward or slow

F80 - F89   Disorders of psychological development

F90 - F98   Behavioural and emotional disorders with onset usually occurring in childhood and adolescence

Unspecified mental disorder
    Mental illness
    Mentally disturbed
    Neuropathy

Appendix B Multiple logistic regression (MLR) and Odds Ratios (OR)

B.1   Interpretation of Odds Ratios

Chapter 1 of this report use logistic regression analysis to provide a measure of the effect of, for example, living in a particular type of institution on having had a particular service or treatment in the past year. Unlike many of the cross tabulations presented elsewhere in the report, MLR estimates the effect of an independent variable while controlling for the confounding effect of other variables in the analysis. A forward stepwise method of logistic regression was used. The dependent variable was binary, indicating the presence or absence of a particular behaviour or state. All variables were categorical.

Logistic regression produces an estimate of the probability of an event occurring when an individual is in a particular category of a socio-demographic variable compared to a reference category of that variable. The odds of the event occurring are defined as the ratio of the probability of the event occurring compared with its absence. If the probability of an event is p, the odds are p/(1-p). The factor by which the odds of an event differ for people in a particular category compared with those in the reference category is shown by the Adjusted Odds Ratio (OR). The OR controls for the possible confounding effects of other variables in the statistical model, eg. sex, age and qualifications. To determine whether the increased odds of the event occurring are due to chance rather than to the effect of the variable, confidence interval associated with the odds ratio are calculated.

B.2   Confidence intervals around an Odds Ratio

In Table 1.21, for example, an odds ratio of 2.08 is shown with a confidence interval from 1.20 to 3.57, indicating that the 'true' (i.e., population) OR is 95% likely to lie between these two values. If the confidence interval does not include 1.00 then the OR is likely to be significantly different from the reference category.

Glossary of survey definitions and terms

Adults

In this survey adults were defined as persons aged 16 or over and less than aged 65.

Antipsychotic drugs

These are also known as 'neuroleptics'. In the short term they are used to quieten disturbed patients whatever the underlying psychopathology.
See Depot Injections

Depot injections

When antipsychotic medication is given by injections on a monthly basis, these are sometimes termed depot injections.

Educational level

Educational level was based on the highest educational qualification obtained and was grouped as follows:

Degree (or degree level qualification)

Teaching, HND, Nursing
    Teaching qualification
    HNC/HND, BEC/TEC Higher, BTEC Higher
    City and Guilds Full Technological
    Certificate
    Nursing qualifications:
    (SRN,SCM,RGN,RM,RHV,
    Midwife)

A level
    GCE A-levels/SCE higher
    ONC/OND/BEC/TEC/not higher
    City and Guilds Advanced/Final level
O level
    GCE O-level (grades A-C if after 1975)
    GCSE (grades A-C)
    CSE (grade 1)
    SCE Ordinary (bands A-C)
    Standard grade (levels 1-3)
    SLC Lower SUPE Lower or Ordinary
    School certificate or Matric
    City and Guilds Craft/Ordinary level

GCSE/CSE
    GCE O-level (grades D-E if after 1975)
    GCSE (grades D-G)
    CSE (grades 2-5)
    SCE Ordinary (bands D-E)

    Standard grade (levels 4-5)
    Clerical or commercial qualifications
    Apprenticeship
    Other qualifications

No qualifications
    CSE ungraded
    No qualifications

Ethnicity

Household members were classified into nine groups by the person answering Schedule A.

White	White
Black - Caribbean	
Black - African	West Indian/African
Black - Other	
Indian	
Pakistani	Asian/Oriental
Bangladeshi	
Chinese	
None of these	Other

For analysis purpose these nine groups were subsumed under 4 headings: White, West Indian/African, Asian/Oriental and Other.

Marital status

Informants were categorised according to their own perception of marital status. Married and cohabiting took priority over other categories. Cohabiting included anyone living together with their partner as a couple.

Physical complaints

Informants were asked 'Do you have any long-standing illness, disability or infirmity? By long-standing I mean anything that has troubled you over a period of time or that is likely to affect you over a period of time?'

Those that answered yes to this question were then asked 'What is the matter with you?'; interviewers were asked to try and obtain a medical diagnosis, or to establish the main symptoms. From these responses, illnesses were coded to the site or system of the body that was affected, using a

classification system that roughly corresponded to
the chapter headings of the International Classification of Diseases (ICD–10). Some of the illnesses
identified were mental illnesses and these were
excluded from the classification of physical illness.
Physical illness did, however, include physical
disabilities and sensory complaints such as eyesight
and hearing problems.

Psychiatric morbidity
The expression psychiatric morbidity refers to the
degree or extent of the prevalence of mental health
problems within a defined area.